RENAL PHYSIOLOGY

NOTICE

Medicine is an ever-changing science. As new research and clinical experience broaden our knowledge, changes in treatment and drug therapy are required.

The author and the publisher of this work have checked with sources believed to be reliable in their efforts to provide information that is complete and generally in accord with the standards accepted at the time of publication. However, in view of the possibility of human error or changes in medical sciences, neither the author nor the publisher nor any other party who has been involved in the preparation or publication of this work warrants that the information contained herein is in every respect accurate or complete. Readers are encouraged to confirm the information contained herein with other sources. For example and in particular, readers are advised to check the product information sheet included in the package of each drug they plan to administer to be certain that the information contained in this book is accurate and that changes have not been made in the recommended dose or in the contraindications for administration. This recommendation is of particular importance in connection with new or infrequently used drugs.

RENAL PHYSIOLOGY

Fourth Edition

Arthur J. Vander, M.D.

Professor of Physiology
University of Michigan

McGRAW-HILL, INC.
Health Professions Division

New York   St. Louis   San Francisco   Colorado Springs
Auckland   Bogotá   Caracas   Hamburg   Lisbon   London   Madrid
Mexico   Milan   Montreal   New Delhi   Paris   San Juan
São Paulo   Singapore   Sydney   Tokyo   Toronto

RENAL PHYSIOLOGY

2 3 4 5 6 7 8 9 0 DOC DOC 9 8 7 6 5 4 3 2 1

This book was set in Times Roman by Better Graphics, Inc.; the editors were
William Day and Lester A. Sheinis; the production supervisor was Clare Stanley.
The cover was designed by Judy Allan.
R. R. Donnelley & Sons Company was printer and binder.

ISBN   0-07-066974-0

Library of Congress Cataloging-in-Publication Data

Vander, Arthur J., date.
   Renal physiology / Arthur J. Vander.—4th ed.
     p. cm.
   Includes bibliographical references.
   Includes index.
   ISBN 0-07-066974-0
   1. Kidneys—Physiology. I. Title.
   [DNLM: 1. Kidney—physiology. WJ 301 V229r]
QP249.V36 1991
612.4'63—dc20
DNLM/DLC
for Library of Congress
                                                90-6417
                                                 CIP

CONTENTS

PREFACE   xi

Chapter 1   FUNCTIONS AND STRUCTURE OF THE KIDNEYS   1
            Objectives   1
            Functions   2
                Regulation of Water and Electrolyte Balance   2
                Excretion of Metabolic Waste Products   3
                Excretion of Foreign Chemicals   3
                Regulation of Arterial Blood Pressure   3
                    The Renin-Angiotensin System   4
                    Other Vasoactive Substances   5
                Secretion of Erythropoietin   5
                Secretion of 1,25-Dihydroxyvitamin D_3 5
                Gluconeogenesis   6
            Structure of the Kidneys and Urinary System   6
                The Nephron   6
                    The Renal Corpuscle   6
                    The Tubule   10
                Blood Supply to the Nephrons   13
                Regional Differences in Structure   15
                The Juxtaglomerular Apparatus   16
                Renal Innervation   16
            Intrarenal Chemical Messengers   17
            Methods in Renal Physiology   17

Chapter 2   BASIC RENAL PROCESSES   19
            Objectives   19
            Glomerular Filtration   23
                Composition of the Filtrate   23

Nature of the Glomerular Barrier
    to Macromolecules   24
Forces Involved in Filtration: Net Filtration
    Pressure   24
Glomerular Filtration Rate (GFR)   26
Tubular Reabsorption   31
Classification of Transport Mechanisms   33
    Diffusion   33
    Facilitated Diffusion   33
    Primary Active Transport   33
    Secondary Active Transport   34
    Endocytosis   34
Transport Mechanisms in Reabsorption   34
Transport Maximum   38
Tubular Secretion   40
Bidirectional Transport   42
Metabolism by the Tubules   43

Chapter 3   RENAL CLEARANCE   44
Objectives   44
Measurement of GFR   44
Definition of Clearance   47
Basic Clearance Formula   48
**Quantitation of Tubular Reabsorption
    and Secretion Using Clearance Methods**   50
**Plasma Creatinine and Urea Concentrations
    as Indicators of GFR Changes**   52

Chapter 4   RENAL HANDLING OF ORGANIC SUBSTANCES   55
Objectives   55
**Glucose, Amino Acids, et al.: Proximal
    Reabsorption of Organic Nutrients**   55
Proteins and Peptides   57
Urea   58
**PAH, Urate, et al.: Proximal Secretion of Organic
    Anions**   61
Proximal Secretion of Organic Cations   63
**Passive Reabsorption or Secretion of Weak
    Organic Acids and Bases**   64

Chapter 5   CONTROL OF RENAL HEMODYNAMICS   68
Objectives   68
Mean Arterial Pressure and Autoregulation   69
Sympathetic Control   73

Angiotensin II   76
  Control of Renin Secretion   77
    Intrarenal Baroreceptors   77
    Macula Densa   77
    Renal Sympathetic Nerves   78
    Angiotensin II   80
    Other Inputs Controlling Renin Release   80
  Prostaglandins   80
  Other Factors   81
  Intrarenal Distribution of Blood Flow   82

**Chapter 6   BASIC RENAL PROCESSES FOR SODIUM,
               CHLORIDE, AND WATER**   83
  Objectives   83
  Sodium Reabsorption and Sodium-Water Coupling   85
  Chloride Reabsorption   89
  Proximal Tubule   90
  Loop of Henle   94
  **Distal Convoluted Tubule and Collecting-Duct
     System**   96
  **Urine Concentration: The Medullary
     Countercurrent System**   99
    Countercurrent Multiplication   100
    The Role of Urea in Maximizing Urine
       Concentration   106
    Countercurrent Exchange: Vasa Recta   106
    Clinical Changes in Urinary Concentrating
       Ability   107
  Summary   109

**Chapter 7   CONTROL OF SODIUM AND WATER
               EXCRETION: REGULATION OF PLASMA
               VOLUME AND OSMOLARITY**   112
  Objectives   112
  Control of GFR   115
    Physiological Regulation of Glomerular-
       Capillary Pressure   115
    Physiological Changes in Plasma Protein
       Concentration   117
    Physiological Control of Glomerular Filtration
       Coefficient (K_f) 117
  Control of Tubular Sodium Reabsorption   118
    Glomerulotubular Balance   118
    Aldosterone   119

Control of Aldosterone Secretion   121
Factors Other Than Aldosterone Influencing
   Tubular Reabsorption of Sodium   122
   Intrarenal Physical Factors: Interstitial
      Hydraulic Pressure   122
   Direct Tubular Effects of Renal Nerves   126
   Direct Tubular Effects of Angiotensin II   126
   Atrial Natriuretic Factor (ANF)
      and Hypothalamic Natriuretic Factor   127
   Other Known Humoral Agents   127
Summary of the Control of Sodium Excretion   128
Abnormal Sodium Retention   129
ADH Secretion and Extracellular Volume   131
ADH and the Renal Regulation of Extracellular
  Osmolarity   133
Thirst and Salt Appetite   135
Summary of the Effects of Angiotensin II   137

Chapter 8   **RENAL REGULATION OF POTASSIUM BALANCE**   139
Objectives   139
Regulation of Internal Potassium Distribution   140
Basic Renal Mechanisms   141
Mechanism of Potassium Secretion in the Cortical
  Collecting Duct   144
Homeostatic Control of Potassium Secretion
  by the Cortical Collecting Duct   145
   Potassium Secretion and Fluid Delivery
      to the Cortical Collecting Duct   149
      Effects of Diuretics   151
The Effects of Acid-Base Changes on Potassium
  Secretion   153

Chapter 9   **RENAL REGULATION OF HYDROGEN-ION**
              BALANCE   155
Objectives   155
Bicarbonate Excretion   159
   Bicarbonate Filtration and Reabsorption   159
   Bicarbonate Secretion   162
Addition of New Bicarbonate to the Plasma (Renal
  Excretion of Acid)   163
   Hydrogen-Ion Secretion and Excretion
      on Urinary Buffers   164
   Phosphate and Organic Acids as Buffers   165
   Qualitative Integration of Bicarbonate
      Reabsorption and Hydrogen-Ion Excretion
      on Nonbicarbonate Buffers   167

Glutamine Catabolism and NH_4^+ Excretion 167
Quantitation of Renal Acid-Base Compensation 169
**Homeostatic Control of Renal Acid-Base
Compensation** 171
Control of Renal Glutamine Metabolism
and NH_4^+ Excretion 171
Control of Tubular Hydrogen-Ion Secretion 172
Specific Categories of Acid-Base Disorders 174
Renal Compensation for Respiratory Acidosis
and Alkalosis 174
Renal Compensation for Metabolic Acidosis
and Alkalosis 175
**Factors Causing the Kidneys to Generate
or Maintain a Metabolic Alkalosis** 176
Influence of Extracellular Volume Contraction 177
Influence of Chloride Depletion 177
Influence of Aldosterone Excess and Potassium
Depletion 178

**Chapter 10   REGULATION OF CALCIUM AND PHOSPHATE
BALANCE** 181
Objectives 181
Effector Sites for Calcium Homeostasis 182
Gastrointestinal Tract 183
Kidneys 183
Bone 184
Hormonal Control of Effector Sites 185
Parathyroid Hormone 185
1,25-Dihydroxyvitamin D_3 188
Calcitonin 189
Other Hormones 189
Overview of Renal Phosphate Handling 189

STUDY QUESTIONS 191

Appendix A.   CLASSES OF DIURETICS 207

**Appendix B.   FIGURES SUMMARIZING ELECTROLYTE
TRANSPORT BY DIFFERENT TUBULAR CELL
TYPES** 208

SUGGESTED READINGS 211

INDEX 221

PREFACE

This book is my attempt to identify the essential core content of renal physiology appropriate for medical students and to present it in a way that permits the student to use the book as his or her primary learning resource. I have been gratified by the wide use the first three editions have achieved and the many letters I have received from medical students (and clinicians) who found that they were, indeed, able to master its contents by independent study.

My major goal in preparing this fourth edition has been to update the material completely but not to alter the level of coverage. Where appropriate, new topics have been added or expanded (atrial natriuretic factor, for example) while the coverage of others has been completely redone because of changes in knowledge. Thus, for example, Chapter 9 has been markedly altered because of our new understanding of bicarbonate secretion and of ammonium production and excretion. I also vowed, however, not to increase the total content of the book, and I'm happy to say that the text is now 5 to 10 percent shorter than the third edition. This was achieved by cutting material not deemed essential. The task of sticking to my intent of presenting only what I consider core material was even more painful this time because of the continued profound expansion of information on renal physiology over the past four years.

My selection of this core material is made explicit in a comprehensive list of behavioral objectives, which tell students specifically what I believe they should know and be able to do by the book's completion. Obviously, no two instructors would come up with exactly the same core material, but it is a simple matter for instructors to give students a supplementary list of objectives to be added or deleted. However, my belief, based on consultations with other physiologists and clinicians, is that these discrepancies are likely to be few. Of much greater importance is the fact that the behavioral objectives (in essence, the content of the book) are explicitly defined so that any such differences are easily determined. This also makes the book quite usable for students in other health sciences, whose required core of information might differ from that of medical students.

In addition to the comprehensive objectives, I have included a large number of study questions with annotated answers. Unlike the lists of objectives, the study questions are neither systematic nor comprehensive in their coverage. Rather, they generally deal with areas I have found to be difficult for students.

Some students profit by using the objectives to guide their readings as they proceed through a chapter. In any case, at the end of each chapter the student should go over the objectives in detail, treating each one as though it were an essay question. Then the student should answer the study questions (at the back of the book) relevant to the chapter. Together, the objectives and study questions provide the means for determining whether the student has mastered the material and for identifying those specific areas that require more work.

The question of how to handle, in an introductory textbook, the enormous emerging complexity of renal physiology is a particularly perplexing one. For so many specific phenomena (for example, sodium reabsorption even within a single tubular segment), there is a multiplicity of processes and controls. To handle this, I have often used the qualifiers ''major'' or ''most important'' in describing those processes included in the book, and I then either simply ignore the others altogether or include them in footnotes. Second, it has gotten to the point where almost every statement of ''fact'' in renal physiology often requires qualification, and I have used footnotes to cite opposing views in certain particularly important controversies. My advice to the student is to ignore the footnotes completely except, of course, in those cases where the instructor feels that material in a footnote is core material. In other words, I have often put into a footnote material that I chose not to include in the text but that, for good reasons, other instructors might feel should be learned by their students.

Another characteristic of this book, like most introductory textbooks, is that it contains almost none of the original research upon which the core of knowledge presented rests. To assure that any interested student can gain entry to this research base as well as pursue any subject in greater depth, I have included an extensive list of Suggested Readings at the back of the book. They are almost all review articles, and their bibliographies provide an entry into the original research literature.

Finally, I have added two appendixes to this edition. The first is a brief summary table of the major types of diuretics, material that is not really ''physiology'' but that, nevertheless, provides a useful review of some of the major concepts concerning renal salt and water handling. The second appendix is a collection of figures illustrating electrolyte handling for each major tubular cell type. Several of these figures also appear in the body of the book, itself, and the essential features of all of them have been described in the text. I decided that their collection in an appendix would make for easy comparison and would make them available for those instructors who feel that they are important for understanding even though all their details need not necessarily be learned by the beginning student.

Arthur J. Vander

1

FUNCTIONS AND STRUCTURE OF THE KIDNEYS

OBJECTIVES

The student states the balance concept.

The student knows the functions of the kidneys.
1 Lists seven functions
2 States the major components of the renin-angiotensin system and their biochemical interrelations
3 Defines inactive prorenin and angiotensin III
4 States the role of erythropoietin

The student defines important gross structures and knows their interrelationships: renal pelvis, calyxes, renal pyramids, medulla (inner and outer), cortex, papilla.

The student understands the interrelationships between the components of a nephron.
1 Defines nephron, renal corpuscle, glomerulus, and tubule
2 Draws the relationship between glomerulus, Bowman's capsule, and the proximal tubule
3 States the three layers separating the lumen of the glomerular capillaries and Bowman's space; defines podocytes, foot processes, slits, and slit diaphragms
4 Defines glomerular mesangium and states its functions
5 Lists in order all the individual tubular segments; states the segments that make up the proximal tubule and the collecting duct system

The student understands the blood supply to the nephron.
1 Lists in order the vessels through which blood flows from renal artery to renal vein
2 Contrasts the blood supply to the cortex and the medulla; defines vasa recta and vascular bundles

The student describes the differences between superficial cortical, midcortical, and juxtamedullary nephrons.

The student defines juxtaglomerular apparatus and describes its three cell types; states the function of the granular cells.

1

The student describes the innervation of the nephron.

The student describes, in general, the renal eicosanoids and the renal kallikrein-kinin system.

FUNCTIONS

The kidneys process blood by removing substances from it and, in a few cases, by adding substances to it. In so doing, they perform the variety of functions summarized in Table 1-1.

Regulation of Water and Electrolyte Balance

The primary function of the kidneys is to balance the body's water and inorganic ions to maintain stable concentrations of these substances in the extracellular fluid, that is, the internal environment. Altering urinary excretion is the means to this balancing end.

Theoretically, a substance can appear in the body either as a result of ingestion or as a product of metabolism. Also, a substance can be excreted from the body or can be metabolized. Therefore, if the quantity of any substance in the body is to be maintained at a constant level over a period of time, the total amounts ingested and produced must equal the total amounts excreted and consumed. This is a general statement of the **balance concept.** For water and hydrogen ion, all four possible pathways apply. However, balance is simpler for the mineral electrolytes. Since they are neither synthesized nor consumed by cells, their total-body balance reflects only ingestion versus excretion.

Reflexes that alter urinary excretion constitute the major mechanisms that regulate the body balances of water and many of the inorganic ions determining the properties of the extracellular fluid. To appreciate the importance of these kidney regulations one need only make a partial list of the more important simple inorganic substances in the internal environment that are regulated, in large part, by the kidneys: water, sodium, potassium, chloride, calcium, magnesium, sulfate, phosphate, and hydrogen ion.

Table 1-1   Functions of the Kidneys

1. Regulation of water and electrolyte balance
2. Removal of metabolic waste products from the blood and their excretion in the urine
3. Removal of foreign chemicals from the blood and their excretion in the urine
4. Regulation of arterial blood pressure by altering both sodium excretion and the secretion of renin and, possibly, other vasoactive substances
5. Secretion of erythropoietin
6. Secretion of 1,25-dihydroxyvitamin D_3
7. Gluconeogenesis

However, the kidneys are not the major regulators of all essential inorganic substances. In particular, the bodily balances of many of the trace elements, such as zinc and iron, are regulated mainly by control of gastrointestinal absorption of the element or by control of biliary secretion. This statement, in large part, is also true of calcium. Nevertheless, even for these elements some renal excretion occurs and may constitute an important source of bodily imbalance in various diseases. Finally, the kidneys also take part in the regulation of some organic nutrients, as will be discussed in subsequent chapters.

Excretion of Metabolic Waste Products

The regulatory role just described is obviously quite different from the popular conception of the kidneys as glorified garbage disposal units that rid the body of assorted wastes and poisons. It is true that some of the chemical reactions that occur within cells result ultimately in end products that must be eliminated. These end products are called waste products because they serve no known biological function in humans. For example, the catabolism of protein produces approximately 30 g of urea per day. Other end products produced in relatively large quantities are uric acid (from nucleic acids), creatinine (from muscle creatine), bilirubin and other end products of hemoglobin breakdown, and the metabolites of various hormones. There are many others, not all of which have been completely identified. Most of these substances are eliminated from the body as rapidly as they are produced, primarily by way of the kidneys. Some of them, e.g., urea, are relatively harmless, but the accumulation of others within the body during periods of renal malfunction accounts for some of the disordered bodily functions in the patient suffering from severe kidney disease. We still are not sure about the identity of these toxins.

Excretion of Foreign Chemicals

The kidneys have another general excretory function, the elimination from the body of many foreign chemicals—drugs, pesticides, food additives, and so on.

Regulation of Arterial Blood Pressure

The kidneys are intimately involved in the regulation of arterial blood pressure through several mechanisms. First, sodium balance is a critical determinant of cardiac output and, possibly, arteriolar resistance over any long time period, and the kidneys, as stated, regulate this balance. Second, the kidneys function as endocrine glands in the **renin-angiotensin system,** a hormonal complex of enzymes, proteins, and peptides that are important in the regulation of arterial pressure (Fig. 1-1).

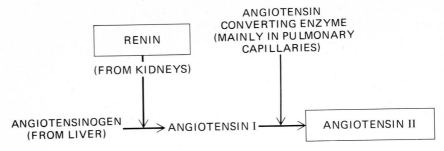

Figure 1-1 Basic biochemistry of the renin-angiotensin system.

The Renin-Angiotensin System **Renin** is a proteolytic enzyme secreted into the blood by the kidneys, specifically by the granular cells of the juxtaglomerular apparatuses (see below). Once in the blood stream, renin catalyzes the splitting of a decapepide, **angiotensin I,** from a plasma protein known as **angiotensinogen,** which is secreted by the liver and is always present in the plasma in high concentration. Under the influence of another enzyme, **angiotensin-converting enzyme,** the terminal two amino acids are then split from the relatively inactive angiotensin I to yield the highly active octapeptide **angiotensin II.** Some converting enzyme is present in plasma, but most is on the endothelial surface of blood vessels, particularly the pulmonary capillaries. Accordingly, the conversion of angiotensin I to angiotensin II occurs mainly as blood flows through the lungs.

  Thus, angiotensin II is a hormone in that it reaches its target organs, including the kidneys, via the arterial blood. However, because the kidneys produce renin and because renal tissue also contains both angiotensinogen and converting enzyme, it is likely that the reactions generating angiotensin I and, in turn, angiotensin II occur to some extent within the kidneys. Accordingly, the kidneys can probably be influenced not only by arterial angiotensin II but also by angiotensin II produced intrarenally.

  As we shall see in subsequent chapters, angiotensin II exerts a large number of effects on diverse tissues, but the end results of most of them are to increase arterial blood pressure. A crucial generalization to be gained from the biochemistry of this system is that because angiotensinogen and converting enzyme are usually present in relatively unchanging concentration, the primary determinant of the rate of angiotensin II formation is the plasma concentration of renin, which is physiologically regulated via the control of renin secretion (to be described in Chap. 5).

  The biochemistry of the renin-angiotensin system is actually far more complex than the description shown in Fig. 1-1. Just a few of the important additional findings are as follows: (1) Approximately half the renin in plasma is the inactive prohormone form of renin **(prorenin)** initially synthesized by the kidneys, and it is possible that this protein can be activated to renin by enzymes in peripheral tissues; (2) renin or reninlike proteins are produced in sites other than the kidneys (e.g., in the uterus and brain) and may catalyze local generation of angiotensin in these sites; (3) clinically important situations exist in which changes in the concentrations of angiotensinogen or converting enzyme occur (e.g., oral contraceptives may cause a large increase in plasma angiotensinogen) and may significantly influence the generation of angiotensin II at any given concentration of renin; and (4) angiotensin II can be split to yield the heptapeptide known as **angiotensin III,** which is also quite active biologically although its relative contribution compared with that of angiotensin II is probably small in most tissues. The enzyme that mediates the generation of angiotensin III is located mainly in the target tissues for this peptide.

Other Vasoactive Substances   In addition to their regulation of salt balance and secretion of renin, the kidneys may exert a third important influence on arterial blood pressure. It is very likely that they either secrete into the blood or remove from it vasoactive substances other than renin. Certainly the kidneys are capable of synthesizing a number of eicosanoids (see below), both vasodilator and vasoconstrictor in action, and the possibility that one or more of these eicosanoids may reach the systemic arterial blood in amounts adequate to dilate or constrict arterioles is the subject of considerable investigation. Secreted vasodilator lipids other than eicosanoids have also been implicated in the renal regulation of arterial blood pressure.

Secretion of Erythropoietin

The kidneys secrete another hormone, **erythropoietin,** which is involved in the control of erythrocyte production by the bone marrow. Just which renal cells secrete erythropoietin is not yet clear, but the stimulus for its secretion is hypoxia in the kidneys (as, for example, in anemia, arterial hypoxia, or inadequate renal blood flow). Erythropoietin stimulates the bone marrow to increase its production of erythrocytes. Erythropoietin will not be described further in this book; it is enough to say that renal disease may result in diminished erythropoietin secretion, and the ensuing decrease in bone marrow activity is one important causal factor in the anemia of chronic renal disease.

Secretion of 1,25-Dihydroxyvitamin D_3

The kidneys produce **1,25-dihydroxyvitamin D_3,** which is the active form of vitamin D. This is the third hormone secreted by the kidneys; its synthesis and role in calcium metabolism will be described in Chap. 10.

Gluconeogenesis

During prolonged fasting, the kidneys synthesize glucose from amino acids and other precursors and release it into the blood. Thus, like the liver, the kidneys are gluconeogenic organs.

STRUCTURE OF THE KIDNEYS AND URINARY SYSTEM

The kidneys are paired organs that lie outside the peritoneal cavity in the posterior abdominal wall, one on each side of the vertebral column. The medial border of the kidney is indented by a deep fissure (called the hilum) through which pass the renal vessels and nerves and in which lies the **renal pelvis,** the funnel-shaped continuation of the upper end of the ureter (Fig. 1-2). The outer convex border of the renal pelvis is divided into major **calyxes,** each of which subdivides into several minor calyxes. Each of the latter is cupped around the projecting apex of a cone-shaped mass of tissue, a **renal pyramid.**

When the kidney is bisected from top to bottom it can be seen to be divided into two major regions: an inner **renal medulla** and an outer **renal cortex.** The medulla is made up of a number of renal pyramids, the apexes of which, as stated in the previous paragraph, project into the minor calyxes. Each apical tip is called a **papilla.** Each pyramid of the medulla, topped by a region of renal cortex, forms a single lobe.

Upon closer gross examination, additional features can be discerned: (1) The cortex has a highly granular appearance, missing from the medulla; (2) each medullary pyramid is divisible into an **outer zone** (adjacent to the cortex) and an **inner zone,** including the papilla. All these distinctions reflect the arrangement of the various components of the microscopic subunits of the kidneys, to which we now turn.

The Nephron

In humans, each kidney is made up of approximately 1 million tiny units termed **nephrons,** one of which is shown diagrammatically in Fig. 1-3. Each nephron consists of a filtering component, called the **renal corpuscle,** and a **tubule** extending out from the renal corpuscle.[1] Let us begin with the renal corpuscle, which is responsible for the initial step in urine formation, the separation of a protein-free filtrate from plasma.

The Renal Corpuscle   The renal corpuscle consists of a compact tuft of interconnected capillary loops, the **glomerulus** (plural = glomeruli),

---

[1] Strictly speaking, the last portions of the tubule, the collecting-duct system, are not part of the nephron, but for simplicity renal physiologists generally ignore this fact, a policy we shall follow.

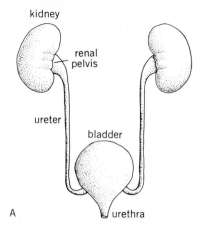

kidney

renal pelvis

ureter

bladder

urethra

A

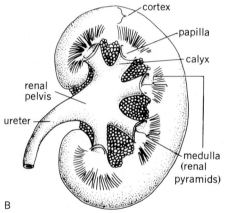

cortex

papilla

calyx

renal pelvis

ureter

medulla (renal pyramids)

B

Figure 1-2 A: The urinary system. The urine formed by a kidney collects in the renal pelvis and then flows through the ureter into the bladder, from which it is eliminated via the urethra. B: Section of a human kidney. Half the kidney has been sliced away. Note that the structure shows regional differences. The outer portion (cortex), which has a granular appearance, contains all the glomeruli. The collecting ducts form a large portion of the inner kidney (medulla), giving it a striped, pyramidlike appearance, and drain into the renal pelvis. The papilla is the inner portion of the medulla.

and a balloonlike hollow capsule, **Bowman's capsule,** into which the glomerulus protrudes (Fig. 1-4).[2] One way of visualizing the relationship between the glomerulus and Bowman's capsule is to imagine a loosely clenched fist (the glomerulus) punched into a balloon (Bowman's capsule). The part of Bowman's capsule in contact with the glomerulus becomes pushed inward but does not make contact with the opposite side of the capsule; accordingly, a space (the **urinary space** or **Bowman's space**) still exists within the capsule, and it is into this space that fluid filters from the glomerulus into Bowman's space.

---

[2] At this point a word about terminology is necessary. Renal physiologists have usually not used the term *renal corpuscle* but rather have used *glomerulus* to denote the combination of capillary tuft and Bowman's capsule and the term *glomerular capillaries* to refer to the tuft. However, a standard nomenclature introduced in 1988 has recommended the usage adopted in this text (see Kriz and Bankir in Suggested Readings). The adjective *glomerular* still denotes events occurring within the renal corpuscle.

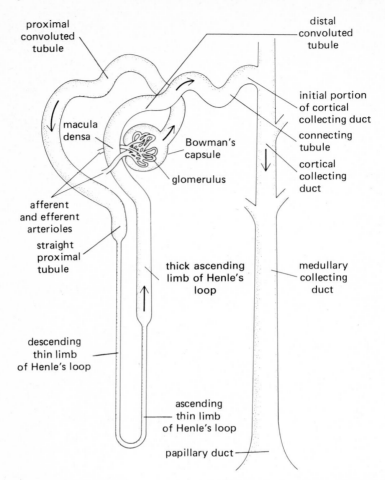

Figure 1-3 Relationships of component parts of a long-looped nephron, which has been "uncoiled" for clarity; relative lengths of the different segments are not drawn to scale. The combination of glomerulus and Bowman's capsule is the renal corpuscle.

The filtration barrier in the renal corpuscle (we shall refer to this barrier as the *glomerular membranes*) consists of three layers: the capillary endothelium of the glomerular capillaries, a basement membrane, and the single-celled layer of epithelial cells constituting Bowman's capsule (Fig. 1-4). The first layer, the endothelial cells of the capillaries, is perforated by many large fenestrae ("windows"). The basement membrane is a relatively homogenous acellular meshwork of glycoproteins and mucopolysaccharides. The capsular epithelial cells that rest on the basement membrane are quite different from the relatively simple, flattened cells that line the rest of Bowman's capsule (the part of the "balloon" not in contact with the "fist") and are called **podocytes.** They have an unusual

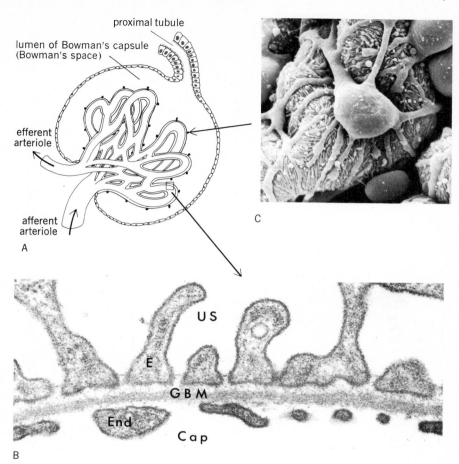

Figure 1-4   A: Anatomy of the renal corpuscle. B. Cross section of glomerular membranes. US = "urinary" (Bowman's) space, E = epithelial foot processes, GBM = glomerular basement membranes, End = capillary endothelium, Cap = lumen of capillary. Note that the basement membrane is itself not homogenous but has a denser core. *(Courtesy HG Rennke; originally published in* Fed Proc *1977; 36:2619; reprinted with permission).* C: Scanning electron micrograph of podocytes covering glomerular capillary loops; the view is from inside Bowman's space. The large mass is a cell body. Note the remarkable interdigitation of the foot processes from adjacent podocytes and the slits between them. *(Courtesy Dr. Craig Tisher.)*

octopuslike structure in that they possess a large number of extensions, or **foot processes,** which are embedded in the basement membrane. The foot processes from adjacent podocytes manifest a great degree of interdigitation. **Slits** exist between adjacent foot processes and constitute the path through which the filtrate, once through the endothelial cells and basement membrane, travels to enter Bowman's space. However, for two reasons, these slits do not offer completely open passageways: (1) The foot processes are coated by a thick layer of extracellular material (glycosialoproteins), which partially occludes the slits; (2) extremely thin diaphragms bridge the slits at the surface of the basement membrane.

The functional significance of this anatomical arrangement is that blood in the glomerulus is separated from Bowman's space by only a thin set of membranes, which permits the filtration of fluid from the capillaries into the space. Bowman's capsule connects, at the side opposite the glomerulus, with the first portion of the tubule, into which this filtered fluid then flows.

Our discussion of the renal corpuscle has focused on the two types of cells—capillary endothelium and podocytes—in the filtration barrier. However, there is a third cell type—**mesangial cells**—found in the central part of the glomerulus between and within capillary loops. Some of the glomerular mesangial cells act as phagocytes, whereas most contain large numbers of myofilaments and are able to contract in response to a variety of stimuli. The role such contraction plays in influencing filtration through the glomeruli will be discussed in Chap. 5.

The Tubule   Throughout its course, the tubule is made up of a single layer of epithelial cells resting on a basement membrane. The structure and function of these epithelial cells vary considerably from segment to segment of the tubule, but one common feature is the presence of tight junctions between adjacent cells.

Physiologists and anatomists have traditionally grouped two or more contiguous tubular segments for purposes of reference, but unfortunately the terminologies used have varied considerably. Table 1-2 lists the names of the various tubular segments (they are illustrated in Fig. 1-5) and

Table 1-2   Terminology for the Tubular Segments

Sequence of segments	Combination terms
Proximal convoluted tubule Proximal straight tubule	Proximal tubule
Descending thin limb of Henle's loop Ascending thin limb of Henle's loop	Intermediate tubule
Thick ascending limb of Henle's loop (contains macula densa near end) Distal convoluted tubule	Distal tubule
Connecting tubule Cortical collecting duct Outer medullary collecting duct Inner medullary collecting duct (last portion is papillary duct)	Collecting-duct system

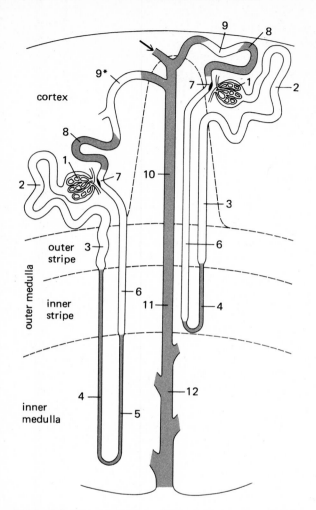

Figure 1-5 Standard nomenclature for structures of the kidney (1988 Commission of the International Union of Physiological Sciences). A short-looped and a long-looped (juxtamedullary) nephron together with the collecting system. Not drawn to scale. A cortical medullary ray—the part of the cortex that contains the straight proximal tubules, cortical thick ascending limbs, and cortical collecting ducts—is delineated by a dashed line. 1, renal corpuscle (Bowman's capsule and the glomerulus); 2, proximal convoluted tubule; 3, proximal straight tubule; 4, descending thin limb; 5, ascending thin limb; 6, thick ascending limb; 7, macula densa (located within the final portion of the thick ascending limb); 8, distal convoluted tubule; 9, connecting tubule; 9*, connecting tubule of a juxtamedullary nephron that arches upward to form a so-called arcade (there are only a few of these in the human kidney); 10, cortical collecting duct; 11, outer medullary collecting duct; 12, inner medullary collecting duct. *(From W Kriz and L Bankir, Am J Physiol 1988; 25:F1-F8; reprinted with permission.)*

combinations recommended by a committee convened in 1988 to standardize nomenclature.

The segment of the tubule that drains Bowman's capsule is the **proximal tubule,** which initially forms several coils (the pars convoluta of the proximal tubule) followed by a straight segment (the pars recta), which descends toward the medulla.

The next segment, into which the proximal straight tubule drains, is the **descending thin limb of Henle's loop** (or simply, the descending loop of Henle). The descending thin limb ends at a hairpin loop, and the tubule then begins to ascend parallel to the descending limb. In long loops (see below), the epithelium of the first portion of this ascending limb remains thin, although different from that of the descending limb, and this segment is called the **ascending thin limb of Henle's loop** (Fig. 1-5). Beyond this segment, in these long loops, the epithelium thickens and this next segment is termed the **thick ascending limb of Henle's loop.** In short loops (see below), there is no ascending thin limb and the thick ascending limb begins right at the hairpin loop (Fig. 1-5).

Near the end of every thick ascending limb, the tubule passes between the arterioles supplying its renal corpuscle of origin (Fig. 1-3). This very short segment—really a plaque in the wall of the thick ascending limb—is known as the **macula densa.** A little beyond the macula densa, the thick ascending limb ends and the **distal convoluted tubule** begins. This is followed by the **connecting tubule,** which leads to a **cortical collecting duct.**

In the great majority of cases, from Bowman's capsule to the ends of the connecting tubules, each of the 1 million tubules in each kidney is completely separate from the others (in a few cases, connecting tubules unite before leading to a cortical collecting duct). The initial portions of approximately 10 cortical collecting ducts then join end to end or side to side to form a single, larger cortical collecting duct. All the cortical collecting ducts then run downward to enter the medulla and become **outer medullary collecting ducts,** and then **inner medullary collecting ducts.** The latter then merge to form several hundred large ducts, the last portions of which are called **papillary collecting ducts,** each of which empties into a calyx of the renal pelvis.

The pelvis is continuous with the **ureter,** which empties into the **urinary bladder,** where urine is temporarily stored and from which it is intermittently eliminated. The urine is not altered after it enters a calyx. From this point on, the remainder of the urinary system simply serves as plumbing.

Table 1-2 lists the names not only of the individual tubular segments but also of the terms presently recommended for denoting multiple consecutive segments: proximal tubule, intermediary tubule, distal tubule, and collecting-duct system. This book will use **proximal tubule** and **collecting-duct system** as defined in the table, but to avoid confusion stemming from other time-honored conventions, it will not refer to *intermediate tubule* or *distal tubule* at all.[3] Also, we will use **loop of Henle** to denote the combination of descending thin limb, ascending thin limb, and thick ascending limb.[4]

As noted earlier, the tubular epithelium is one-cell thick throughout. Until the distal convoluted tubule, the cells in any given segment are homogenous and distinct for that segment. Thus, for example, the ascending thick limb contains only "ascending thick limb cells." However, beginning late in the distal convoluted tubule, several cell types may intermingle within a given segment. Moreover, these cell types may exist, in different proportions, in the various segments. The two most important such cell types in the collecting ducts are the **principal cells** and the **intercalated cells.** The principal cells are the more numerous type.

Blood Supply to the Nephrons

In the earlier section on the renal corpuscle, we described the glomerular capillaries but made no mention of the origin of these capillaries. Blood enters each kidney via a renal artery, which then divides into progressively smaller branches—interlobar, arcuate, and finally cortical radial (formerly interlobular) arteries. Each of the cortical radial arteries gives off at right angles to itself, as it courses toward the kidney surface, a parallel series of **afferent arterioles** (Figs. 1-3 and 1-6), each of which leads to a glomerulus. (Thus, the afferent arteriole is the "arm" to which the "fist" is attached.)

Normally, only about 20 percent of the plasma (and none of the erythrocytes) entering the glomerulus is filtered from the capillaries into Bowman's capsule. Where does the remaining blood go next? In almost all other organs, capillaries recombine to form the beginnings of the venous system. The glomerular capillaries instead recombine to form another set of arterioles called the **efferent arterioles.** Thus, blood leaves each glomerulus through a single efferent arteriole (Fig. 1-4), which soon subdivides into a second set of capillaries (Fig. 1-6). These **peritubular capillaries** are profusely distributed to, and intimately associated with, all the portions of the tubule, an arrangement that permits movement of solutes and water between the tubular lumen and capillaries. The peritubular capillaries then rejoin to form the veins by which blood ultimately leaves the kidney.

[3] Physiologists have previously used *distal tubule* to denote not the structures in Table 1-2 but the combination of the distal convoluted tubule, connecting tubule, and initial portion of the cortical collecting duct. In this usage, the distal convoluted tubule was called *early distal tubule* and the other structures *late distal tubule*. (See Kriz and Bankir in Suggested Readings.)

[4] The anatomists' *loop of Henle* denotes not this combination but rather the combination of the proximal straight tubule, descending thin limb, and ascending thin and thick limbs, the last segment often called the *distal straight tubule*. (See Kriz and Bankir in Suggested Readings.)

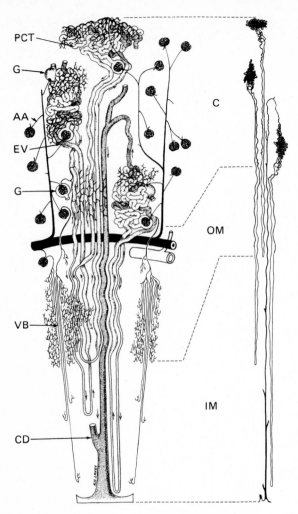

Figure 1-6 Diagram of renal vascular and tubular organization. Only three nephrons (one from each general population) are shown, vascular structures are extensively simplified, and vertical scale is compressed. The same nephrons are shown undistorted to the right. Major zones are cortex (C), outer medulla (OM), and inner medulla (IM). Afferent arterioles (AA), glomeruli (G), and efferent vessels (EV) are shown together with part of the peritubular capillary network. The proximal convoluted tubules (PCT) and distal convoluted tubules (dark hatching) are generally dissociated from the efferent network arising from their parent glomeruli. Some midcortical efferents directly perfuse loops of Henle and collecting ducts in cortical medullary rays. In outer medulla, descending thin limbs of short loops are close to vascular bundles (VB), and thin limbs of long loops are found with thick ascending limbs and collecting ducts (CD) in the interbundle region. Note the relationships of the capillary plexuses (CP) to the vascular bundles. (*Courtesy Reiner Beeuwks III; adapted from* Am J Physiol, *1975; 229:695.*)

In general, both the efferent arteriole from a given glomerulus and the peritubular capillaries arising from that arteriole are dissociated from the tubule originating from that glomerulus; i.e., the efferent arteriole supplies a different tubule. Moreover, the various segments of any single tubule are supplied with blood coming from multiple efferent arterioles.

Regional Differences in Structure

There are important regional differences in the locations of the various tubular and vascular components. The cortex contains all the renal corpuscles (this accounts for its granular appearance), convoluted portions of the proximal tubule, cortical portions of Henle's loops, distal convoluted tubules, connecting tubules, and cortical collecting ducts.

Nephrons are categorized according to the locations of their glomeruli in the cortex (Fig. 1-5): (1) In **superficial cortical nephrons** glomeruli are located within 1 mm of the capsular surface of the kidneys; (2) in **midcortical nephrons** glomeruli are located, as their name states, in the midcortex, deep to the superficial cortical nephrons but above the next category; (3) in **juxtamedullary nephrons** glomeruli are located just above the corticomedullary junction. One major distinction among these three categories is the length of the loop of Henle. All superficial cortical nephrons have short loops of Henle, which make their turn superficial to the junction of outer and inner medulla. All juxtamedullary nephrons have long loops, which extend into the inner medulla, often to the tip of a papilla. Midcortical nephrons may be either short-looped or long-looped. The additional length of the loop of Henle in long-looped nephrons is due entirely to the length of the thin segments. Finally, the beginning of the thick ascending limb in the longest loops marks the border between outer and inner medulla.

The three nephron populations differ from each other structurally in ways other than the lengths of their loops of Henle. Moreover, the midcortical nephrons themselves are not homogenous but manifest gradations of structural characteristics as one moves inward. All this structural heterogeneity is reflected in functional heterogeneity.

The vascular structures supplying the medulla also differ from those in the cortex (Fig. 1-6). From many of the juxtamedullary glomeruli, long efferent arterioles extend to the outer medulla, where they divide many times to form **vascular bundles.** The margins of these bundles give rise to a capillary network that surrounds loops of Henle and collecting ducts in the outer medulla. From the cores of the bundles, straight vessels (**descending vasa recta**) extend to the inner medulla, where they break up into a capillary plexus. These inner medullary capillaries re-form into veins (**ascending vasa recta**) that run in close association with the descending vasa recta within the vascular bundles. This relationship, as we shall see, has considerable significance for the formation of concentrated urine.

The Juxtaglomerular Apparatus

Reference was made earlier to the macula densa, that portion of the late thick ascending limb that in all nephrons courses between the afferent and efferent arterioles at the hilus of the glomerulus of its own nephron. This entire area is known as the **juxtaglomerular (JG) apparatus** (Fig. 1-7). (Don't confuse the term *juxtaglomerular apparatus* with *juxtamedullary nephron.*) Each JG apparatus is made up of three cell types: (1) **granular cells,** which are differentiated smooth muscle cells in the walls of the arterioles, particularly in the afferent arterioles; (2) extraglomerular mesangial cells; and (3) macula densa cells.

The granular cells (so-called because they contain secretory vesicles) are the cells that secrete the hormone renin, mentioned earlier in this chapter. The extraglomerular mesangial cells are morphologically similar to and continuous with the intraglomerular mesangial cells described earlier, but their function is unknown. The mascula densa is in contact with the vascular component of the juxtaglomerular apparatus, and the macula densa cells contribute both to the control of renin secretion (Chap. 7) and to the control of glomerular filtration rate (Chap. 5).

Renal Innervation

The kidneys receive a rich supply of sympathetic noradrenergic neurons. These are distributed to the afferent and efferent arterioles, the juxtaglomerular apparatus, and many portions of the tubule. There is no

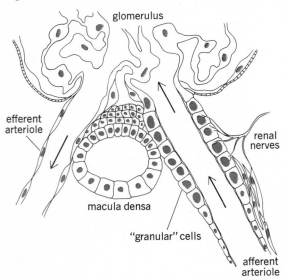

Figure 1-7 Diagram of a glomerulus showing the juxtaglomerular apparatus. The granular cells secrete renin and are also thought to function as baroreceptors. Mesangial cells are not shown. (*Redrawn from JO Davis,* Am J Med 1973; 55:333.)

significant parasympathetic innervation. There are some dopamine-containing neurons, the functions of which are unknown.

INTRARENAL CHEMICAL MESSENGERS

As we shall see in subsequent chapters, the kidneys are the target organs for multiple neural and hormonal inputs. In addition, in response to appropriate stimuli, the kidneys themselves synthesize a variety of substances that function as intrarenal chemical messengers. The biochemistry of several of these will be described briefly here, and their postulated functions will be dealt with in subsequent chapters.

As pointed out earlier, intrarenally generated angiotensin II is one such substance. So are the eicosanoids. The glomerular endothelium and all the tubular segments, the medullary collecting ducts being the predominant site, produce **PGE$_2$**. Although PGE$_2$ is the major renal eicosanoid, the kidneys also can produce others, including PGF$_{2a}$, PGD$_2$, thromboxane A$_2$, and prostacyclin.

A third group of intrarenally generated chemical messengers is the **kinins,** the collective name given to **lysyl bradykinin** and **bradykinin.** The kinins are peptides released from plasma protein precursors—kininogens—by several plasma and tissue enzymes called **kallikreins.** The specific kallikrein produced and secreted by the kidneys splits plasma kininogen to yield lysyl bradykinin, which is cleaved again within the kidneys to yield bradykinin (note the analogies between the kallikrein-kinin and renin-angiotensin systems).

One of the most fascinating (and confusing) features of the renin-angiotensin system, the renal eicosanoids, and the renal kallikrein-kinin system is the host of interactions being discovered among these three groups of chemical messengers. Only those interactions considered best established and important will be described in subsequent chapters, but the interested reader may obtain more information by consulting the Suggested Readings.

Finally, these three complex groups by no means exhaust the list of likely intrarenal chemical messengers, and several others will be mentioned later.

METHODS IN RENAL PHYSIOLOGY

Because of its limited scope and objectives, this book will deal very little with the methods used to study renal physiology. Only the method known as *clearance* is described to an extent (in Chap. 3) because of its widespread clinical use. Another technique that has been a mainstay of renal physiologists is **micropuncture,** the insertion of a micropipette into a nephron segment to withdraw fluid for analysis as well as to measure pressures, perfuse tubules, and perform other manipulations on single nephrons in situ. A third technique is that of perfusing isolated separated segments of a single nephron in vitro, and this has made possible many studies that could not be done with older techniques. For example, micropuncture is generally applicable only to the most superficial nephrons since these can be visualized by looking down on the surface of the kidney. This had been a major impediment to studying medullary structures and functional heterogeneity of nephrons.

In addition to clearance, micropuncture, and the isolated, perfused tubule, a plethora of other useful techniques has been developed, and all of them, like the "big three," have particular advantages and disadvantages. The interested reader should consult the Suggested Readings at the back of the book.

Study questions: 1 and 2

2

BASIC RENAL PROCESSES

OBJECTIVES

The student knows the basic principles of renal physiology.

 1 Lists and defines the three basic renal processes: glomerular filtration, tubular reabsorption, tubular secretion
 2 Describes the routes for blood and fluid movements within the kidneys
 3 Describes the composition of the glomerular filtrate; describes glomerular "sieving"
 4 States the sites in the glomerular membranes for restriction of macromolecules; defines steric hindrance and electrical hindrance and relates them to protein filtration
 5 States the formula for the determinants of glomerular net filtration pressure and gives normal values
 6 States the factors determining glomerular filtration rate; defines hydraulic permeability and filtration coefficient (K_f)
 7 States how mesangial cells alter K_f
 8 Describes how arterial pressure, afferent-arteriolar resistance, and efferent-arteriolar resistance determine glomerular-capillary pressure
 9 States the effect of obstruction on P_{BC}.
10 Describes the determinants of π_{GC} and how the rate of plasma flow influences this variable
11 Predicts the direction of change of GFR under a variety of situations, including hypotension, reduced plasma protein concentration, and ureteral occlusion
12 Defines and states the major characteristics of diffusion, facilitated diffusion, primary active transport, secondary active transport, and endocytosis
13 States how the mechanisms of Objective 12 can be combined to achieve reabsorption or secretion
14 Defines the concept of T_m (either reabsorptive or secretory); given appropriate data, calculates T_m; defines threshold; defines splay; states the significance of a T_m being much higher than the usual filtered mass of the substance
15 Defines pump-leak system and states its consequences
16 Contrasts "tight" and "leaky" epithelia

Urine formation begins with **glomerular filtration,** the bulk-flow of essentially protein-free plasma from the glomerular capillaries into Bowman's capsule. The final urine that enters the renal pelvis is quite different from this **glomerular filtrate** because, as the filtrate flows from Bowman's capsule through the various portions of the tubule, its composition is altered. This change occurs through two general processes: tubular reabsorption and tubular secretion. The tubule is at all points intimately associated with the peritubular capillaries, a relationship that permits transfer of materials between the peritubular-capillary plasma and the lumen of the tubule. When the direction of transfer is from tubular lumen to peritubular-capillary plasma, the process is called **tubular reabsorption.** Movement in the opposite direction, i.e., from peritubular-capillary plasma to tubular lumen, is called **tubular secretion.** This last term must not be confused with **excretion.** To say that a substance has been excreted is to say that it appears in the final urine. These relationships are illustrated in Fig. 2-1.

The most common relationships among these basic renal processes—glomerular filtration, tubular reabsorption, and tubular secretion—are shown in the hypothetical examples of Fig. 2-2. Plasma, containing three low-molecular-weight substances, X, Y, and Z, enters the glomerular

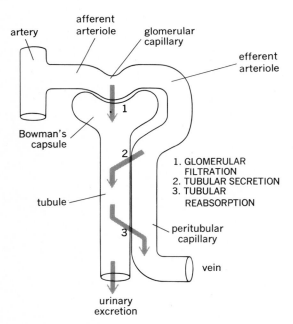

Figure 2-1 The three basic components of renal function. *(From AJ Vander et al.,* Human Physiology, *New York, McGraw-Hill, 1990.)*

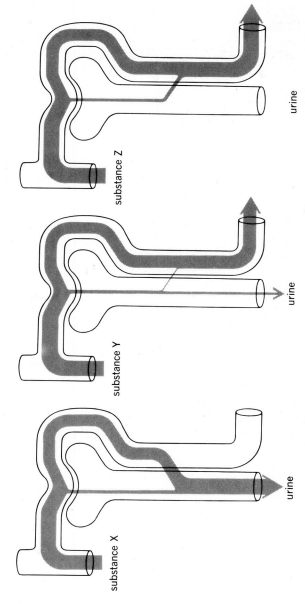

Figure 2-2 Renal manipulation of three hypothetical substances, X, Y, and Z. X is filtered and secreted but not reabsorbed. Y is filtered, and a fraction is then reabsorbed. Z is filtered but is completely reabsorbed. *(From AJ Vander et al., Human Physiology. New York, McGraw-Hill, 1990.)*

capillaries, and approximately 20 percent of the plasma is filtered into Bowman's capsule. The filtrate, which contains X, Y, and Z in the same concentrations as the plasma remaining in the capillaries, enters the proximal convoluted tubule and begins its flow through the rest of the tubule. Simultaneously, the remaining 80 per cent of the plasma, with its X, Y, and Z, leaves the glomerular capillaries via the efferent arterioles and enters the peritubular capilliaries. The cells of the tubular epithelium can secrete all the peritubular-capillary X into the tubular lumen but cannot reabsorb X. Thus, by the combination of filtration and tubular secretion, all the plasma that originally entered the renal artery is cleared of substance X, which leaves the body via the urine. The tubule can also reabsorb Y and Z. The amount of Y reabsorption is small, so most of the filtered Y is not reabsorbed and escapes from the body in the urine. But for Z the reabsorptive mechanism is so powerful that virtually all the filtered Z is reabsorbed back into the plasma. Therefore, no Z is lost from the body. Hence, the processes of filtration and reabsorption have canceled each other, and the net result is as though Z had never entered the kidney at all.

The kidneys work only on plasma. The erythrocytes supply oxygen to the kidneys but serve no other function in urine formation.

For each plasma substance, a particular combination of filtration, reabsorption, and secretion applies. The critical point is that the rates at which the relevant basic processes proceed for many of these substances are subject to physiological control. What is the effect, for example, if the filtered mass of Y is increased or its reabsorption rate decreased? Either change causes more Y to be lost from the body via the urine. By triggering changes in the rates of filtration, reabsorption, or secretion whenever the plasma concentration of a substance goes above or below normal, homeostatic mechanisms can regulate the substance's plasma concentration.

In summary, one can study the normal renal handling of any given substance by asking a series of questions:

1   To what degree is the substance filterable at the glomerulus?

2   Is it reabsorbed?

3   Is it secreted?

4   What are the mechanisms by which reabsorption or secretion is achieved?

5   What factors homeostatically regulate the quantities filtered, reabsorbed, or secreted, i.e., what are the pathways by which renal excretion of the substance is altered to maintain stable body balance?

6   What factors other than renal disease can perturb body balance by causing the kidneys to filter, reabsorb, or secrete too much or too little of the substance?

For clinicians, of course, a seventh question must be asked: How do the various types of renal disease influence the handling of the substance and its total-body balance?

GLOMERULAR FILTRATION

Composition of the Filtrate

The glomerular membranes (this term includes all three components of the filtration barrier in the renal corpuscle) are freely permeable to water and to **crystalloids,** i.e., solutes of small molecular dimensions. They are relatively impermeable to large molecules, or **colloids,** the most important of which are the plasma proteins. Therefore, the glomerular filtrate, i.e., the fluid within Bowman's capsule, is essentially protein-free and contains crystalloids in virtually the same concentrations as in the plasma.[1] The only exceptions to the last part of this generalization are certain crystalloids that would otherwise be filterable but are partially bound to plasma proteins; the protein-bound moiety does not filter out of the capillary. For such a substance, the concentration in Bowman's capsule will equal not the full plasma concentration but the plasma concentration of the substance not bound to protein. For example, 40 percent of the plasma calcium is protein-bound, and so the calcium concentration of the glomerular filtrate is 60 percent of that in plasma.

We must point out the reason for use of the phrase "essentially protein-free" in the previous paragraph. In reality, the glomerular filtrate does contain extremely small quantities of protein (almost entirely albumin), on the order of 10 mg/L or less. This is about 0.02 percent of the concentration of protein in plasma. This protein crosses the glomerular membranes to reach Bowman's space by both bulk-flow along with the other components of the filtrate and by simple diffusion. In various disease states, the glomerular membranes may be altered to permit marked increases in the passage of protein into Bowman's space. Moreover, even in the absence of glomerular-membrane alteration, when certain small proteins not normally present in the plasma appear because of disease (e.g., hemoglobin released from damaged erythrocytes, and myoglobin released from damaged muscles), considerable filtration of them may occur.

This occurrence emphasizes that the glomerular membranes behave as all-or-none filters only with regard to crystalloids and very large pro-

---

[1] Actually, the concentrations of charged crystalloids in Bowman's capsule are not exactly the same as in plasma water because the plasma proteins cause a Donnan equilibrium to exist between these fluids. This effect is small, however, and may be ignored.

teins. There is no hindrance to the movement of molecules with molecular weights less than 7000 and essentially total hindrance to molecules the size of plasma albumin; for molecules between these extremes, fil- terability becomes progressively smaller. This is known as **sieving.**

Nature of the Glomerular Barrier to Macromolecules

The route that filtered substances take through the glomerular membranes is as follows: fenestra in the endothelial layer, basement membrane, slit diaphragms, and slits. Most of the restriction to macromolecules takes place in the basement membrane, in the hydrated spaces between the elongated, intertwining glycoprotein chains constituting this gel-like layer. However, restriction by this primary filter is not absolute for most macromolecules, and some that do traverse the entire thickness of the basement membrane encounter futher restriction both by the slit di- aphragms and by the coats of the podocytes, which occupy much of the slits. (This is a good time to reread the glomerular anatomy section of Chap. 1.) The reader might well wonder what happens to macromolecules that get hung up at these sites; they are probably taken into the foot processes by endocytosis and broken down.

The discussion thus far has dealt only with steric hindrance, i.e., impairment of macromolecular movement solely because of size. How- ever, electric charge is also a critical variable in determining penetration by proteins and other macromolecules. The molecules that constitute the glomerular barrier's extracellular matrix (the cell coats of the endo- thelium, the basement membrane, and the cell coats of the podocytes) are almost all polyanions. Accordingly, for any given size, negatively charged macromolecules are restricted more than neutral molecules are from entering and moving through the barrier because the fixed polyanions repel the negatively charged molecules. (It is useful to imagine simply that the route followed constitutes "pores" lined with negative charges.) Since almost all proteins bear net negative charges, this electrical hin- drance plays an important restrictive role, enhancing that of purely steric hindrance. It is very likely that many of the diseases that cause renal corpuscles to be "leaky" to protein do so by eliminating many of the negative charges in the wall.

It must be emphasized that these negative charges act as a hindrance only to macromolecules, not to the plasma crystalloids, which are too small to be significantly influenced by any charges "lining the pores."

Forces Involved in Filtration: Net Filtration Pressure

The **net filtration pressure (NFP)** for any capillary is the algebraic sum of the opposing hydraulic (also called hydrostatic) and colloid osmotic (oncotic) pressures acting across the capillary. This also applies to the glomerular capillaries:

$$\text{NFP} = \underbrace{(P_{GC} + \pi_{BC})}_{\text{forces inducing filtration}} - \underbrace{(P_{BC} + \pi_{GC})}_{\text{forces opposing filtration}}$$

where P_{GC} = glomerular-capillary hydraulic pressure
   π_{BC} = oncotic pressure of fluid in Bowman's capsule
   P_{BC} = hydraulic pressure in Bowman's capsule
   π_{GC} = oncotic pressure in glomerular-capillary plasma

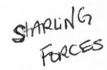

STARLING FORCES

Because there is virtually no protein in Bowman's capsule, π_{BC} may be taken as zero, and the equation becomes (Fig. 2-3)

$$\text{NFP} = P_{GC} - P_{BC} - \pi_{GC}$$

The hydraulic pressures in glomerular capillaries and Bowman's capsule have not been directly measured in people. However, several lines of indirect evidence suggest that the human values are probably similar to those for the dog, and the latter are shown in Table 2-1 and Fig. 2-4 along with glomerular capillary oncotic pressure.

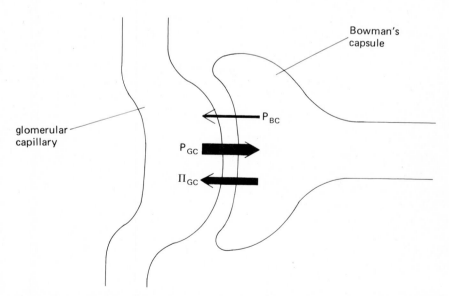

Figure 2-3 Net filtration pressure in the renal corpuscle equals glomerular-capillary hydraulic pressure (P_{GC}) minus Bowman's capsule hydraulic pressure (P_{BC}) minus glomerular-capillary oncotic pressure (π_{GC}).

Table 2-1   Forces Involved in Glomerular Filtration in Dogs

	mmHg	
Forces	Afferent end of glomerular capillary	Efferent end of glomerular capillary
1 Favoring filtration: Glomerular-capillary hydraulic pressure, P_{GC}	60	58
2 Opposing filtration: a Hydraulic pressure in Bowman's capsule, P_{BC}	15	15
b Oncotic pressure in glomerular capillary π_{GC}	21	33
3 Net filtration pressure (1 − 2)	24	10

Note that both the hydraulic and oncotic pressures in the glomerular capillaries change along the length of the capillaries: (1) Capillary hydraulic pressure decreases slightly because of the resistance to flow offered by the capillaries; (2) oncotic pressure increases because, since the filtrate is essentially protein-free, the filtration process removes water but not protein from the plasma, thereby increasing the protein concentration and, hence, the oncotic pressure of the unfiltered plasma remaining in the glomerular capillaries.[2]

Figure 2-4 and Table 2-1 show that in the dog, net filtration pressure is 24 mmHg at the beginning of the glomerular capillaries and 10 mmHg at the end. As stated above, these values are probably a reasonable approximation of those for normal human beings.[3]

Glomerular Filtration Rate (GFR)

The volume of filtration from glomerular capillaries into Bowman's capsule per unit time is known as the **glomerular filtration rate (GFR).** The GFR depends not only on the net filtration pressure (NFP) described in

---

[2] For physiochemical reasons we will not discuss, the relationship between oncotic pressure and plasma protein concentration is not linear. Oncotic pressure increases proportionally more than plasma protein concentration at protein concentrations greater than those of normal plasma.

[3] However, because this is by no means a certainty, it should at least be noted that in all species of experimental animals directly studied, other than the dog, glomerular-capillary hydraulic pressure normally is lower than the value observed in dogs. Therefore, net filtration pressure is also lower and may actually become zero at some point along the glomerular capillary, a phenomenon known as filtration pressure equilibrium. This situation may also occur in human beings when glomerular-capillary pressure is unusually low, as for example, following a severe hemorrhage. Why the existence of filtration pressure equilibrium is important is given in the next two footnotes. (See Brenner and Humes, and Deen et al., in Suggested Readings.)

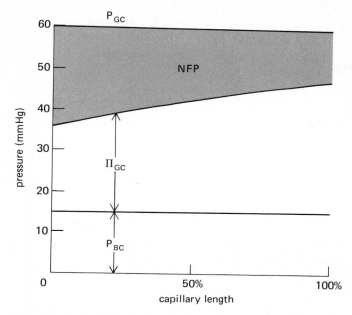

Figure 2-4 Glomerular filtration pressures in dog. Net filtration pressure (NFP) = P_{GC} − π_{GC} − P_{BC}. It is likely that values for human beings are similar to those of the dog, except under certain pathological conditions.

the previous section but also on both the hydraulic (water) permeability of the glomerular membranes and the surface area available for filtration:

GFR = hydraulic permeability × surface area × NFP

The product of hydraulic permeability and surface area is known as the **filtration coefficient (K_f)**. Accordingly,

$$\text{GFR} = K_f \times \text{NFP}$$

Let us expand the equation to reemphasize all of its components

$$\text{GFR} = \underset{\substack{\text{(hydraulic permeability)} \\ \times \text{ surface area)}}}{K_f} \times \underset{(P_{GC} - P_{BC} - \pi_{GC})}{\text{NFP}}$$

In a normal 70-kg person, the GFR is 180 L/day (125 mL/min)! Contrast this figure with the net filtration of fluid across all the other capillaries in the body—approximately 4 L/day. That a net filtration pressure of approximately 10 to 24 mmHg suffices to filter this huge volume of fluid is attributable to the fact that K_f for glomerular capillaries

Table 2-2   Summary of Direct GFR Determinants and Factors That Influence
Them

Direct determinants of GFR: GFR = $K_f(P_{GC} - P_{BC} - \pi_{GC})$	Major factors that tend to increase the magnitude of the direct determinant
K_f*	(1) ↑ glomerular surface area because of relaxation of glomerular mesangial cells Result: ↑ GFR
P_{GC}*	(1) ↑ renal arterial pressure (2) ↓ afferent-arteriolar resistance (afferent dilation) (3) ↑ efferent-arteriolar resistance (efferent constriction) Result: ↑ GFR
P_{BC}*	(1) ↑ intratubular pressure because of obstruction of tubule or extrarenal urinary system Result: ↓ GFR
π_{GC}*	(1) ↑ systemic-plasma oncotic pressure (sets π_{GC} at beginning of glomerular capillaries) (2) ↓ total renal plasma flow (sets rate of rise of π_{GC} along glomerular capillaries) Result: ↓ GFR

*K_f = filtration coefficient; P_{GC} = glomerular-capillary hydraulic pressure; P_{BC} = Bowman's capsule hydraulic pressure; π_{GC} = glomerular-capillary oncotic pressure. A reversal of all arrows in the table will cause a decrease in the magnitudes of K_f, P_{GC}, P_{BC}, and π_{GC}.

relative to nonrenal capillaries is very large. The reasons are that the glomerular capillaries have a large surface area, but more important, they have a much greater (10–100 fold) hydraulic permeability.

The implications of this huge GFR are extremely important. When we recall that the average total volume of plasma in humans is approximately 3 L, it follows that the entire plasma volume is filtered by the kidneys some 60 times a day. The opportunity to process such huge volumes of plasma enables the kidneys to excrete large quantities of waste products and to regulate the constituents of the internal environment very precisely.

The GFR is not fixed but may show marked fluctuations in differing physiological states and in disease. If all other factors remain constant, any change in K_f, P_{GC}, P_{BC}, or π_{GC} will alter GFR. The next question becomes: What factors influence these direct determinants of GFR (Table 2-2)?

K_f   Changes in K_f can occur in glomerular disease, but this variable is also subject to physiological control. A variety of chemical mediators causes contraction of glomerular mesangial cells, with a resulting de-

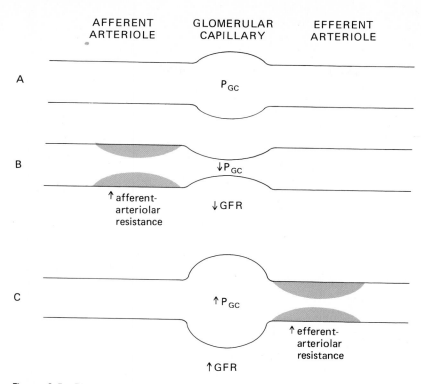

Figure 2-5 Effects of pure afferent-arteriolar constriction (B) or pure efferent-arteriolar constriction (C) on P_{GC} and, hence, GFR.

crease in glomerular surface area and, hence, K_f. This decrease in K_f will tend to lower GFR.[4]

P_{GC} Glomerular-capillary hydraulic pressure (P_{GC}) is the determinant of GFR under tightest physiological control. P_{GC} reflects the interplay of renal arterial pressure, afferent-arteriolar resistance (R_A), and efferent-arteriolar resistance (R_E). As should be clear from Fig. 2-5, a change in renal arterial pressure will *tend* to cause a change in P_{GC} of the same direction. (As will be described in Chap. 5, the phrase "tend to cause"

---

[4] Why the phrase "tend to" in this sentence? The basic equation relating K_f and GFR predicts that any decrease in K_f should definitely cause a directly proportional decrease in GFR. However, this prediction does not apply to GFR under conditions in which filtration pressure equilibrium (footnote 3) occurs well before the end of the glomerular capillaries. Under this condition, filtration, although reduced proportionally to K_f at every locus along the length of the capillary, will continue beyond the point in the capillary at which filtration pressure equilibrium previously had occurred. In this way, the total volume filtered along the entire length of capillary may change little, if at all. (See Brenner and Humes, and Deen et al., in Suggested Readings.)

here and elsewhere in this discussion reflects the fact that other simultaneously occurring events may oppose the effect of the specific factor being analyzed.) At any given renal arterial pressure, an increase in R_A (afferent-arteriolar constriction) will tend to lower P_{GC}, simply by causing a greater loss of pressure between the renal arteries and glomerular capillaries. Conversely, a decrease in R_A (afferent-arteriolar dilation) will tend to raise P_{GC}. More difficult to visualize is the fact that changes in R_E also tend to cause changes in P_{GC}, changes opposite to those caused by changes in R_A. Thus, an increase in R_E (efferent-arteriolar constriction) tends to elevate P_{GC}. This occurs because the efferent arteriole lies beyond the glomerulus, so that efferent-arteriolar constriction tends to "dam back" the blood in the glomerular capillaries, raising P_{GC}. Similarly, a decrease in R_E (efferent-arteriolar dilation) tends to lower P_{GC}.

P_{BC} The major cause of increased hydraulic pressure in Bowman's capsule is obstruction anywhere along the tubule or in the external portions of the urinary system (e.g., ureter). The effect of such an occlusion is to increase the tubular pressure everywhere proximal to the occlusion, all the way back to Bowman's capsule. The result is to decrease GFR.

π_{GC} Oncotic pressure in the plasma at the very beginning of the glomerular capillaries is, of course, simply the oncotic pressure of systemic arterial plasma. Accordingly, a decrease in systemic plasma protein concentration, as occurs, for example, in liver disease, will lower arterial oncotic pressure and tend to increase GFR, whereas increased arterial oncotic pressure will tend to reduce GFR.

But now recall (Fig. 2-4 and Table 2-1) that π_{GC} is identical to systemic plasma oncotic pressure *only* at the very beginning of the glomerular capillaries and that π_{GC} then progressively increases along the glomerular capillaries as protein-free fluid filters out of the capillary, concentrating the protein left behind. As we have seen, this means that net filtration pressure and, hence, GFR progressively decrease along the capillary length. Accordingly, anything that favors a steeper rise in π_{GC} will tend to lower total GFR. This is what occurs when total renal plasma flow is low; it shouldn't be hard to visualize that the initial filtration of a given volume of fluid from a small total volume of plasma flowing through the glomeruli will cause the protein left behind to become more concentrated than if the total volume of plasma were quite large. In other words, the presence of a low rate of total plasma flow through the glomeruli, all other factors being constant, will cause π_{GC} to rise more steeply.[5]

[5] Thus, there is a potential automatic link between total renal plasma flow and GFR, an increase or decrease in the former tending to cause an automatic change of similar direction in the latter. However, although conclusive data are not available, this automatic link between renal plasma flow and GFR is probably not a very important one, quantitatively, in human beings under most physiological conditions since it applies mainly when filtration pressure equilibrium is achieved (footnotes 3 and 4).

Summary   Table 2-2 presents a summary of the material described in this section. It provides, in essence, a checklist of questions to ask when trying to ascertain why GFR has changed in any particular situation. First, which of the *direct* determinants of GFR is responsible for the change in GFR? Second, what factor is responsible for the change in this direct determinant? Finally, and not shown in the table, the normal physiological inputs (nerves, hormones, etc.) regulating these latter factors will be described in Chaps. 5 and 7.

TUBULAR REABSORPTION

Many filterable plasma components are either completely absent from the urine or present in smaller quantities than were originally filtered at the renal corpuscle. This fact alone is sufficient to prove that these substances undergo tubular reabsorption. An idea of the magnitude and importance of these reabsorptive mechanisms can be gained from Table 2-3, which summarizes data for a few plasma components that undergo filtration and reabsorption. The values in Table 2-3 are typical for a normal person on an average diet. There are at least three important generalizations to be drawn from this table:

   1   The filtered quantities are enormous, generally larger than the amounts of the substances in the body. For example, the body contains about 40 L of water, but the volume of water filtered each day is 180 L. If reabsorption of water ceased but filtration continued, the total plasma water would be urinated within 30 min.
   2   Reabsorption of waste products such as urea is relatively incomplete, so that large fractions of their filtered amounts are excreted in the urine.
   3   Reabsorption of most "useful" plasma components, e.g., water, electrolytes, and glucose, is relatively complete, so that the amounts excreted in the urine represent very small fractions of the filtered amounts.

Table 2-3   Average Values for Several Substances
Handled by Filtration and Reabsorption

Substance	Amount filtered per day	Amount excreted	% reabsorbed
Water, L	180	1.8	99.0
Sodium, g	630	3.2	99.5
Glucose, g	180	0	100
Urea,* g	56	28	50

*Handling of urea is actually more complicated than just filtration and reabsorption (see Chap. 4).

With regard to generalization 3, an important distinction should be made between reabsorptive processes that can be controlled physiologically and those that cannot. The reabsorption rates of many organic nutrients, for example, glucose, are always very high relative to the quantities filtered and are not physiologically regulated. Therefore, the filtered amounts of these substances are normally *completely* reabsorbed, none appearing in the urine. For these substances, like substance Z in our earlier example, it is as though the kidneys did not exist because the kidneys do not normally eliminate them from the body at all. Therefore, the kidneys do not help *regulate* the plasma concentrations of these substances, i.e., minimize changes from their operating points. Rather, the kidneys merely maintain whatever plasma concentrations already exist, generally the result of hormonal regulation of nutrient metabolism.

In contrast, the reabsorption rates for water and many ions, although also very high, are regulatable. Consider what happens when a person drinks a lot of water: Within 1 to 2 h all the excess water has been excreted in the urine, chiefly, as we shall see, as the result of decreased renal-tubular reabsorption of water. In this example, the kidney is the effector organ of a reflex that maintains plasma water concentration within very narrow limits. The critical point is that in contrast to those for glucose, the rates at which water and the inorganic ions are reabsorbed and, therefore, the rates at which they are excreted are subject to physiological control.

It is essential to realize that tubular reabsorption is a process fundamentally different from glomerular filtration. The latter occurs completely by bulk-flow, in which water and all dissolved free (non-protein-bound) crystalloids move together. In contrast, there is relatively little bulk-flow across the tubular-epithelial cells from lumen to interstitium because there are few, if any, hydraulic and oncotic pressure gradients and because the tubular epithelium is relatively much less porous than the glomerular membranes. (Recall that tubular-epithelial cells are joined together by tight junctions.) It must be emphasized that we are speaking here only of the relative lack of bulk-flow from tubular lumen to interstitium; as will be seen later, there is bulk-flow from interstitial fluid into peritubular capillaries, and this constitutes one of the ways (diffusion being the other) for a reabsorbed substance, having made it from tubular lumen to interstitial fluid, to complete its journey by gaining entry to the peritubular capillaries.

What are the mechanisms for reabsorption? The reabsorption of some substances occurs through diffusion, whereas that of others requires more or less discrete transport processes. The phrase "more or less discrete" denotes two important facts: (1) The reabsorption of different substances may be linked (e.g., the reabsorption of many amino acids, glucose, and other solutes is linked to that of sodium); (2) a single reabsorptive system may be capable of transporting several distinct, but structurally similar, substances (e.g., at least four of the simple carbohydrates are reabsorbed by a single system).

The transport mechanisms involved in tubular reabsorption are basically the same mechanisms involved in membrane transport anywhere in the body.

Classification of Transport Mechanisms

Diffusion This process arises from random molecular motion and requires an electrochemical gradient for net movement to occur; i.e., net diffusion is always "downhill." Lipid-soluble substances can diffuse across a cell's plasma membranes, whereas ionic diffusion is restricted pretty much to water-filled channels created by the arrangement of the plasma-membrane's proteins. These channels may be highly specific for certain ions; thus, we speak of "sodium channels" or "potassium channels."

Facilitated Diffusion This process, like diffusion, can produce net movement of a subtance only down its electrochemical gradient (thus, the term *diffusion*). However, unlike simple diffusion, the transport depends on interaction of the substance with specific membrane proteins, which "facilitate" its movements. This is one important mechanism for accelerating the movement of non-lipid-soluble molecules, and the membrane proteins involved are termed carriers. The initial event in facilitated diffusion is the binding of the substance to be transported to the carrier, followed by a conformational change in the carrier that causes the transported substance's translocation across the membrane. The substance then separates from the carrier. Because of the interaction with membrane proteins, facilitated diffusion manifests specificity, saturability, and competition.

Primary Active Transport In this process, the transported molecule also interacts with membrane proteins (carriers) and exhibits specificity, saturability, and competition. In contrast to facilitated diffusion, however, primary active transport produces net uphill transport, i.e., net transport against an electrochemical gradient. The energy for this active transport comes directly from the splitting of ATP. Indeed, the term *primary* specifically denotes that metabolically produced chemical energy is the direct source of the energy for the process. In such cases, membrane-bound ATPase not only splits the ATP to provide energy but also is a component of the actual carrier mechanism. Presently documented primary active transporters are the Na,K-ATPase, H-ATPase, H,K-ATPase, and Ca-ATPase.

Secondary Active Transport (Cotransport and Countertransport)   In this process, two (or sometimes more) substances interact simultaneously with the same specific membrane proteins (carriers), and both are translocated across the membrane. The crucial point is that one of the substances undergoes only net "downhill" transport (facilitated diffusion), whereas the other manifests net "uphill" movement against its electrochemical gradient. Yet, the latter occurs without input of metabolic energy *directly* into the transport process. Rather, the direct source of energy is the energy liberated by the simultaneous downhill facilitated diffusion of the other transported substance. In other words, as one of the substances (often sodium) moves down its electrochemical gradient, the energy released somehow is able to drive the other substance uphill against its electrochemical gradient. The substance moving uphill is said to undergo **secondary active transport** because the active transport is not directly linked to ATP hydrolysis the way primary active transport is.

The term **cotransport** denotes the situation in which the involved substances are moving in the same direction across the membrane, one downhill and the other uphill. In **countertransport** the energy liberated by the downhill movement of one of the substances produces uphill movement of the second substance in the *opposite* direction. For example, the downhill movement of sodium *into* the cell might provide the energy for uphill movement of hydrogen ion *out of* the cell.

Endocytosis   This process is characterized by the invagination of a portion of the plasma membrane until it becomes completely pinched off and exists as an isolated intracellular membrane-bound vesicle filled with the extracellular fluid it imbibed during its formation. This process offers an important mechanism for the uptake of macromolecules, which may trigger off the entire process by binding to specific membrane proteins. Endocytosis, of course, requires energy, and its source is the splitting of ATP. Thus endocytosis is technically a form of primary active transport.

Transport Mechanisms in Reabsorption

We began this discussion of tubular reabsorptive mechanisms with the statement that they are simply the basic mechanisms for transport across any plasma membranes, but we must now face the added complexity that arises when one deals with an epithelial layer, such as the renal tubule (or gastrointestinal epithelium, gallbladder epithelium, etc.), rather than the plasma membrane of a single nonepithelial cell (a muscle cell or erythrocyte, for example).

Look at Fig. 2-6 and you will see that there are two potential routes for reabsorptive movement from lumen to interstitium. The first is by diffusion *between* cells, i.e., across the tight junctions connecting cells, and is termed **paracellular**. Paracellular reabsorption requires that an

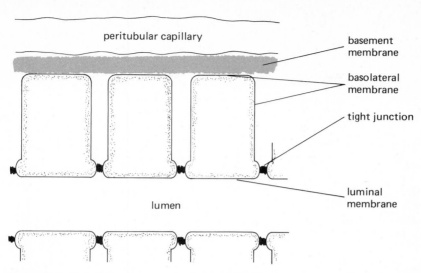

Figure 2-6 Diagrammatic representation of tubular epithelium. The tight junctions can be visualized three-dimensionally as the sheet of plastic holding together a six-pack of beer, each cell being one of the cans.

electrochemical gradient exist for the substance in the reabsorptive direction and that the tight junctions are permeable to the substance. We shall describe in later chapters how such electrochemical gradients are created across the tubule for various substances.

The second route is **transcellular** ("across" the cell), in which the reabsorbed substance must cross *two* plasma membranes in its journey from tubular lumen to interstitial fluid—the **luminal** (or apical) **membrane** (separating the luminal fluid from the cell cytoplasm) and the **basolateral membrane** (separating the cytoplasm from the interstitial fluid).

Accordingly, to fully characterize the overall transport of a substance across the epithelium, one must know whether paracellular transport exists and, for transcellular transport, what characteristics exist for the luminal membrane and the basolateral membrane. (The basement membrane, on which the epithelial layer rests, must also be traversed, but because it serves only a structural role and is not a significant barrier to the movement of solutes or water, we shall ignore it. For this reason it will not be shown in subsequent figures illustrating either reabsorptive or secretory processes.)

Let us take sodium reabsorption in the cortical collecting ducts as an example. The first question is whether paracellular reabsorption occurs for sodium in this tubular segment. The answer is *yes,* but this process is quite minor and we will ignore it now and deal only with the much more important transcellular reabsorption of sodium, illustrated in Fig. 2-7. Sodium ions move downhill across the luminal membrane into the

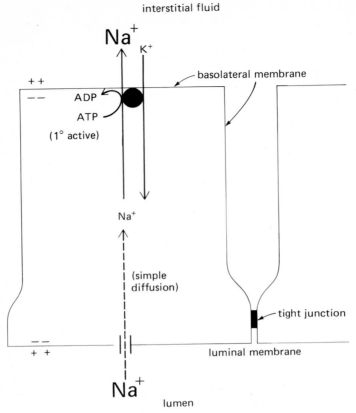

interstitial fluid

Figure 2-7 Reabsorption of sodium in the cortical collecting duct. Diffusion into the cell through the sodium channels in the luminal membrane is driven by the sodium concentration gradient (cytosolic sodium being much lower than luminal sodium) and the potential difference (cytosol negative relative to lumen), both ultimately the result of the basolateral primary active Na, K-ATPase "pumps." In this tubular segment, the potassium ions actively transported into the cell by the pumps diffuse out through channels in both the luminal and basolateral membranes (see Chap. 8); these paths are not shown in the figure in order to focus on only the sodium.

cytoplasm through channels. The sodium ions are then actively transported across the basolateral membrane into the interstitial fluid. This latter "pump" is a primary active process that involves Na,K-ATPase, found only in the basolateral membranes. Thus, the unidirectional reabsorptive movement of sodium is made possible by the asymmetry of the luminal and basolateral membranes.

What may not be apparent from this brief description is the fact that the luminal and basolateral events do not occur in isolation from each other. This becomes evident as soon as one recognizes that the net diffusion of sodium across the luminal membrane depends on the existence of a favorable electrochemical gradient—cytoplasmic [Na] < lumi-

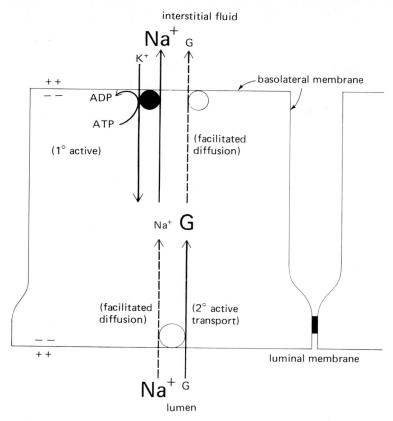

Figure 2-8 "Secondary active reabsorption" of glucose by the proximal tubule. Follow this figure by beginning with the primary active Na pump in the basolateral membrane. Then you will see how the low intracellular sodium concentration and intracellular negativity permit the net downhill entry of sodium across the luminal membrane, which in turn provides the energy for simultaneous uphill glucose movement across this membrane. Luminal glucose concentration is shown falling toward zero as it is reabsorbed.

nal [Na] and electric potential oriented so that the cell interior is negative relative to the lumen. The crucial point is that the basolateral Na,K-ATPase pump creates this electrochemical gradient across the luminal membrane by keeping the cytoplasmic [Na] low and the cell interior negatively charged. The role of the pump in the creation of intracellular negativity need not be dealt with here.

Let us take another example, the reabsorption of glucose (Fig. 2-8), which occurs in the proximal tubule. Glucose moves from the lumen across the luminal membrane into the cytoplasm by cotransport with sodium. This carrier-mediated movement of glucose is secondary active transport since the energy utilized to drive the uphill movement of glucose across the luminal membrane is derived from the simultaneous downhill movement of sodium. So efficient is this uphill movement that the lumen can be virtually cleared of glucose. After entry into the cell, the glucose then exits across the basolateral membrane by facilitated diffusion, this downhill movement being driven by the high-glucose concentration achieved in the cell by the action of the luminal transport process.

A critial point, easy to miss, is that the entire overall process of glucose reabsorption depends ultimately on the primary active Na,K-ATPase pump in the basolateral membrane. Only because of this pump is the electrochemical gradient maintained for net facilitated diffusion of sodium across the luminal membrane, and it is this downhill process that provides the energy for the simultaneous uphill movement of the glucose. Now the reader should be able to understand why glucose reabsorption is termed secondary active transport—it is itself uphill ("active") but is "secondary" to (dependent on) "primary" active transport of sodium. Instead of glucose, we could have used amino acids, phosphate, or a variety of organic substances as our example, for they, too, undergo secondary active reabsorption by being cotransported with sodium in precisely the same manner.

One more note about terminology: When referring to transcellular transport, the term *active* is a shorthand way of stating that at least one of the two membrane crossings is achieved by a primary or secondary active process, i.e., that uphill transport against the substance's electrochemical gradient has occurred somewhere between lumen and interstitial fluid. Thus, we say that glucose undergoes active reabsorption.

Finally, it is worth stating again that we have so far dealt only with the movement of substances from tubular lumen to interstitium. The final step in reabsorption is movement from interstitium into peritubular capillaries. This step, for all reabsorbed substances, occurs by bulk-flow and/or diffusion and will be described in Chap. 6.

Transport Maximum

Many of the active reabsorptive systems in the renal tubule have a limit, termed a **transport maximun** (T_m), to the amounts of material they can transport per unit time because the membrane proteins responsible for the transport become saturated. An important example is the secondary active transport process for glucose in the proximal tubule. Normal persons do not excrete glucose in their urine because all filtered glucose is reabsorbed, but it is possible to produce urinary excretion of glucose in a completely normal person merely by administering large quantities of glucose directly into a vein (Table 2-4).

Note in Table 2-4 that even after the plasma glucose concentration and, hence, the filtered quantity of glucose has doubled, the urine is still glucose-free, indicating that the T_m for reabsorbing glucose has not yet been reached. But as the plasma glucose and the filtered load continue to

Table 2-4   Experimental Data Obtained for Calculation of Glucose T_m

Time, min	GFR, mL/min	P_G, mg/mL	Filtered glucose (GFR × P_G), mg/min	Excreted glucose ($U_G V$),* mg/min	Reabsorbed glucose (filtered − excreted), mg/min
0	125	1.0	125	0	125
Begin glucose infusion					
26–40	125	2.0	250	0	250
100–110	125	4.0	500	125	375
130–140	125	5.0	625	250	375

*U_G = urine concentration of glucose; V = urine volume per time.

rise, glucose finally appears in the urine because all the filtered glucose cannot be reabsorbed. Once the T_m for glucose, which equals 375 mg/min, has been exceeded, any further increase in plasma glucose is accompanied by a proportionate increase in excreted glucose. The tubules are now reabsorbing all the glucose they can, and any amount filtered in excess of this quantity cannot be reabsorbed and appears in the urine. This is what occurs in patients with diabetes mellitus. Because of a deficiency in pancreatic production of insulin, the patient's plasma glucose may rise to extremely high values. The filtered load of glucose becomes great enough to exceed T_m, and glucose appears in the urine. There is nothing wrong with the tubular transport mechanism for glucose. It is simply unable to reabsorb the huge filtered load.

To add one more level of complexity, let us return to the experiment in which glucose was infused. Additional data were obtained for minutes 60 to 100 but were not shown in Table 2-4. They are as follows:

Time, min	GFR, mL/min	P_G mg/mL	Filtered glucose, mg/min	Excreted glucose, mg/min	Reabsorbed glucose, mg/min
60–80	125	2.8	350	20	330
80–100	125	3.5	436	76	360

Now we see that glucose began to be excreted in the urine *before* the true T_m of 375 mg/min was reached. The plasma concentration at which glucose first appears in the urine is known as the **threshold** for glucose. The appearance of glucose in the urine before the T_m is reached is termed **splay.** There are two reasons for splay: (1) A carrier-mediated mechanism shows kinetics analogous to those of enzyme systems, so that maximal activity is substrate-dependent (in this case, glucose-dependent); i.e., the pump may not work at its absolute maximal rate until the luminal glucose concentration is too high to permit all of it to be "captured" by the pump. (2) Not all nephrons have the same T_m for glucose, so that some may be spilling glucose at a time when others have not yet reached their T_ms. This last point is important, for we too often fall into the habit of viewing the kidneys as one large nephron. The fact is that there are really more than 2 million nephrons in the kidneys, and they are not identical in functional characteristics.

Except for our experimental subject who received intravenous glucose, the plasma glucose in normal persons never becomes high enough to cause urinary excretion of glucose because the T_m for glucose is much greater than necessary for normal filtered loads. However, for certain other substances, the reabsorptive T_m is very close to the normal filtered load, sometimes already in the splay portion of the reabsorptive pattern. Therefore, even a small increase in the plasma concentration of such a substance would produce large increases in its excretion.

TUBULAR SECRETION
Tubular secretory processes transport substances across the tubular epithelium into the lumen, i.e., in the direction opposite to tubular reabsorption, and constitute a second pathway into the tubule, the first pathway being glomerular filtration.

The overall secretory process for any given substance begins with its diffusion out of the peritubular capillaries into the interstitial fluid, from which it makes its way into the lumen by crossing either the tight junctions—the paracellular route—or, in turn, the basolateral and luminal membranes of the cell—the transcellular route. As is the case for reabsorption, paracellular secretory movement requires a favoring electrochemical gradient for the substance and permeability of the tight junctions to the substance. In the case of transcellular secretion, the net secretory movement results from differences in the characteristics of the two membranes. For example (Fig. 2-9), the secreted substance might be pumped across the basolateral membrane by a primary or secondary active process, and the resulting high intracellular concentration could then drive movement across the luminal membrane by diffusion or facilitated diffusion. Of course, positioning of the active secretory step on the luminal membrane and the passive step on the basolateral membrane would achieve the same final result, i.e., net movement into the tubular lumen. As is true for tubular reabsorption, the overall process of tubular secretion can be categorized as active or passive depending on whether an uphill process occurs across at least at one of the membranes.

Since the first step in the active secretion of a substance is diffusion of the substance from peritubular capillary into interstitial fluid, you might suppose that substances mainly bound to plasma proteins could not

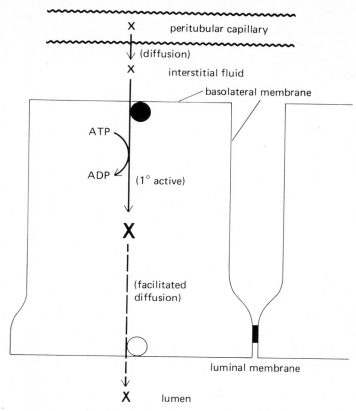

Figure 2-9 Secretory pathway for hypothetical substance X.

undergo tubular secretion. However, such is not the case. There are always some free molecules of the substance in equilibrium with those bound to plasma proteins, and as the free molecules diffuse out of the capillary, others come off the plasma proteins, by mass action, to take their place. This happens rapidly enough so that in those cases in which a secretory system exists for a protein-bound substance, almost all the substance originally bound to the protein can still undergo secretion, often during a single passage of blood through the kidneys.

Among the most important secretory processes are those for hydrogen ion and potassium, and these will be discussed in detail later. (As an appetizer, go back to Fig. 2-7 and simply insert a potassium channel in the luminal membrane so that some of the potassium entering across the basolateral membrane via the Na,K-ATPase pumps can exit across the luminal membrane; *voilà*, this cell now not only actively reabsorbs sodium but also actively secretes potassium.)

There are also, in the proximal tubule, several low-specificity secretory systems for organic anions and cations (Chap. 4).

BIDIRECTIONAL TRANSPORT

In the preceding sections, the adjective *net* was frequently used in reference to tubular reabsorption or secretion and was always implicit even
when absent. The fact is that only rarely, if ever, does any transported
substance manifest purely unidirectional flux across the tubule totally
unopposed by a flux in the other direction.

One important reason for bidirectional transport is apparent from
reconsideration of the example in Fig. 2-9. Note that because of the
primary active transport process in the basolateral membrane, the overall
secretory process achieves a concentration higher in the lumen than in the
interstitial fluid. This difference, of course, favors a net movement in the
reabsorptive direction by diffusion so that if the tight junctions or plasma
membranes are at all permeable to substance X, such movement will
occur. Similarly, active reabsorptive processes tend to establish a concentration lower in the lumen than in the interstitial fluid, and this concentration difference favors passive secretion.

Thus, we are dealing with so-called **pump-leak systems,** in which the
active pump creates a diffusion gradient that opposes its own action by
favoring back-diffusion. Since this back-diffusion occurs solely as an
indirect result of the pump's activity and since the *net* flux will, therefore,
always be in the direction of the pump, we do not usually dignify the back-
diffusion with the terms *reabsorption* or *secretion*. In other words, in
reference to Fig. 2-9, we say simply that X is handled by secretion, and we
do not call the passive back-flux *reabsorption*. To take the sodium pattern
of Fig. 2-7 as another example, we say simply that sodium is reabsorbed,
and we do not assign the term *secretion* to the passive back-flux into the
lumen.

The "leak" component of epithelial pump-leak systems is a very
important determinant of the maximal concentration gradients that can be
established across the epithelial layer. Thus, to refer again to Fig. 2-9, the
more permeable the epithelium is to X, the more difficult it will be for the
secretory mechanisms (the "pump") to increase luminal X concentration
above interstitial-fluid X concentration. Similarly, an active reabsorptive
mechanism is less able to lower the luminal concentration of the transported substance below its interstitial-fluid concentration when the permeability of the epithelial layer to that substance is very high.

For most mineral ions and many organic molecules, the major route
for the "leak" in pump-leak systems is paracellular. On the basis of the
relative permeability of the tight junctions, as manifested by their electrical resistances, various epithelia are classified as "leaky" or "tight."
Leaky epithelia include the proximal tubules (as well as the epithelia of

the small intestine and gallbladder). Tight epithelia include the distal convoluted tubules and collecting ducts.

To reiterate, leaky epithelia do not achieve large ionic concentration gradients between lumen and interstitial fluid. In addition, only relatively low electrical potentials exist across them (because the passive leak "short-circuits" the potentials), and they have high water permeabilities. In contrast, tight epithelia can exhibit large concentration differences between tubular lumen and interstitium, large transcellular potential differences, and low water permeabilities. These characteristics should be kept in mind when we discuss, in subsequent chapters, the transport of ions and water by the proximal (leaky) and more distal (tight) segments of the tubule.

Pump-leak systems are not the only cause of bidirectional transport within a single tubular segment. Another reason is that a nephron segment may contain either opposing pathways, often residing in distinct cell types in the segment, or "reversible pumps" for a particular substance. The nephron segment may, therefore, manifest net secretion or net reabsorption, depending on the physiological circumstances.

Finally, for many substances, a given tubular segment may always manifest only reabsorption or only secretion, but other tubular segments may do just the opposite. For example, a substance may be secreted into the proximal tubule but reabsorbed from the collecting duct. In such cases, the relative magnitudes of the opposing processes in the different tubular segments determine whether the overall effect of the entire tubule will be reabsorption or secretion.

METABOLISM BY THE TUBULES

Although renal physiologists have traditionally listed glomerular filtration, tubular reabsorption, and tubular secretion as the three basic renal processes, a fourth process—metabolism by the tubular cells—is also of considerable importance for many substances. For example, the tubular cells may extract organic nutrients from the peritubular capillaries, but rather than secreting them into the lumen, the cells may metabolize them as dictated by the cells' own nutrient requirements. In so doing, the renal cells are behaving no differently than any other cells in the body.

In contrast, other metabolic transformations performed by the kidney are not directed toward its own nutritional requirements but rather toward altering the composition of the urine and plasma. The most important of these are the synthesis of ammonium from glutamine and the production of bicarbonate, both described in Chap. 9.

Study questions: 3 to 12

3

RENAL CLEARANCE

OBJECTIVES
The student understands the principles and applications of clearance technique.
1   Defines the term *clearance*
2   States the criteria that must be met for a substance for its clearance to be used as a measure of GFR: states which substances are used to measure GFR and ERPF
3   Lists the data required for clearance calculation
4   Given data, calculates $C_{In}, C_{PAH}, C_{urea}, C_{glucose}, C_{Na}$
5   Predicts whether a substance undergoes net reabsorption or net secretion by comparison of its clearance to that of inulin, or by comparison of its rate of filtration to its rate of excretion.
6   Given data, calculates net rate of reabsorption or secretion for any substance
7   Given data, calculates reabsorptive T_m for glucose and secretory T_m for PAH
8   Given data, calculates fractional excretion of any substance
9   Knows how to estimate GFR from C_{urea} and describes the limitations
10 Describes the limitation of C_{Cr} as a measure of GFR
11 Constructs the curve relating steady-state P_{Cr} to C_{Cr} or P_{urea} to C_{urea}; predicts the changes in P_{Cr} and P_{urea} given a known change in GFR: knows the limitations of this analysis, particularly with regard to urea

The technique known as *clearance* is extremely useful for evaluating renal function. Before defining it and developing it in a more formal manner, we shall look at an example of how it is used—the measurement of glomerular filtration rate.

MEASUREMENT OF GFR
Assume there is a substance (let us call it W) that is freely filterable at the renal corpuscle but neither secreted nor reabsorbed by the tubules. Then,

$$\frac{\text{Mass of } W \text{ excreted}}{\text{Time}} = \frac{\text{Mass of } W \text{ filtered}}{\text{Time}} \qquad (3\text{-}1)$$

44

Since the mass of any solute equals the product of solute concentration and solvent volume,

$$\frac{\text{Mass of } W \text{ excreted}}{\text{Time}} = \frac{\text{urine conc of } W \times \text{urine volume}}{\text{Time}} \qquad (3\text{-}2)$$

Conc = $\dfrac{\text{mass}}{\text{vol.}}$

Combining Eqs. (3-1) and (3-2),

$$U_W V = \frac{\text{Mass of } W \text{ filtered}}{\text{Time}} \qquad (3\text{-}3)$$

where U_W = urine concentration of W
$ V$ = urine volume per unit time

so $\dfrac{\text{amt. in urine}}{\text{time}} = \dfrac{\text{amt. filtered}}{\text{time}}$

Of course, the mass of W filtered also equals the product of the volume of plasma filtered into Bowman's capsule and the concentration of W in the filtrate. The volume of plasma filtered per unit time is, by definition, the glomerular filtration rate (GFR). Since W is freely filterable, the filtrate concentration of W is the same as the arterial plasma concentration P_W. Therefore,

$$\frac{\text{Mass of } W \text{ filtered}}{\text{Time}} = P_W \times \text{GFR} \qquad (3\text{-}4)$$

Combining Eqs. (3-3) and (3-4),

$\underline{P_W \times \text{GFR} = \text{amt. in plasma}}$

$$U_W V = P_W \times \text{GFR} \qquad (3\text{-}5)$$

Three of the variables—V, P_W, and U_W—can be measured, and we can solve for GFR:

$$\text{GFR} = \frac{U_W V}{P_W} \qquad = \frac{\text{amt. of } W \text{ in urine}}{\text{conc. of } W \text{ in plasma}} \qquad (3\text{-}6)$$

The validity of the above analysis depends on the following characteristics of W:

1 Freely filterable at the glomerulus
2 Not reabsorbed
3 Not secreted
4 Not synthesized by the tubules
5 Not broken down by the tubules

A polysaccharide called **inulin** (not insulin) completely fits this description and can be used for the determination of GFR. Consider the following hypothetical situation: To determine your patient's GFR, you infuse inulin at a rate sufficient to maintain plasma concentration constant at 4 mg/L. Urine collected over a 2-h period has a volume of 0.2 L and an inulin concentration of 360 mg/L. What is the patient's GFR?

$$GFR = \frac{U_{In}V}{P_{In}}$$

$$GFR = \frac{360 \text{ mg/L} \times 0.2 \text{ L/2 h}}{4 \text{ mg/L}}$$

$$GFR = 18 \text{ L/2 h} = 9 \text{ L/h}$$

If any of the five criteria listed above were not valid for inulin, its use would not provide an accurate measure of GFR. For example, if inulin were secreted, which of the following statements would be true?

Calculated GFR would be higher than the true GFR.
Calculated GFR would be lower than the true GRF.

The first statement is correct because the mass of inulin excreted (the numerator in the GFR equation) would represent both filtered and secreted inulin and, therefore, would be greater than the filtered inulin.

Unfortunately, measuring GFR with inulin is inconvenient because inulin is not a normally occurring bodily substance and must be administered intravenously at a continuous constant rate for several hours. Therefore, in clinical situations the endogenous substance **creatinine** is frequently used to *estimate* GFR. Creatinine is formed from muscle creatine and released into the blood at a fairly constant rate. Consequently, its blood concentration changes little during a 24-h period, so that one need obtain only a single blood sample and a 24-h urine collection.

$$\text{Estimated GFR} = \frac{U_{Cr}V}{P_{Cr}}$$

This is only an estimated GFR because, in humans, creatinine does not meet all five criteria since it is secreted by the tubules. It therefore overestimates the true GFR. However, because the amount secreted is relatively small, the discrepancy is not very large.[1] In a later section we will describe how measurement of plasma creatinine alone without any urine determinations can also be used to estimate GFR more crudely. Use of urea for the same purpose will also be described.

---

[1] Unfortunately, the discrepancy does become large when GFR is very low because secreted creatinine then becomes a significant fraction of excreted creatinine.

DEFINITION OF CLEARANCE

When we described how inulin could be used to measure GFR, we were actually describing the technique known as clearance. First, let us define the term. The **clearance** of a substance is the *volume of plasma* from which that substance is *completely cleared* by the kidneys *per unit time*. Every substance in the blood has its own distinct clearance value, and the units are always in volume of plasma per time. Inulin offers an excellent example. Since all excreted inulin must come from the plasma, one can see that a certain volume of plasma loses its inulin while flowing through the kidney; i.e., a certain volume of plasma is "cleared" of inulin. For inulin, this volume is obviously equal to the GFR since none of the inulin contained in the glomerular filtrate returns to the blood (inulin is not reabsorbed) and since none of the plasma that escapes filtration loses any of its inulin (inulin is not secreted). Therefore, a volume of plasma equal to the GFR has been completely cleared of inulin. This volume is termed the inulin clearance and is expressed as C_{In}. Accordingly,

$$C_{In} = GFR$$

What is the glucose clearance? Glucose is freely filtered at the renal corpuscle so that all the glucose contained in the glomerular filtrate is lost *initially* from the plasma to the tubules. But all this filtered glucose is then normally reabsorbed; i.e., it is all returned to the plasma. The net result is that *no* plasma ends up losing glucose; the clearance of glucose is *zero*.

Let us take another example—phosphate (for the purposes of this example, we will assume that plasma phosphate, P_{PO_4}, is completely filterable). Here are some normal data:

GFR = 180 L/day
P_{PO_4} = 1 mmol/L
$U_{PO_4}V$ = 20 mmol/day

Clearance = how much plasma must be completely cleared of its PO_4 to supply 20mmol/day to urine.

What is the phosphate clearance in this example? The filtered phosphate equals 180 mmol/day. Is this the phosphate clearance? The answer is no. Clearance does *not* designate a filtered mass. Indeed, it does not designate any mass; it is always a volume per time. The clearance of phosphate is defined as the volume of plasma completely cleared of phosphate per unit time. Is the clearance of phosphate, then, the GFR? Again the answer is no. Certainly, the filtered phosphate contained in the GFR is *initially* lost from the plasma, but much of it is reabsorbed, in this example, 160 mmol/day, leaving only 20 mmol/day to be excreted in the urine. Is this the phosphate clearance?

Once again the answer is *no*. Clearance is not defined as mass excreted but rather as the volume of plasma supplying that mass per unit time. In other words, the phosphate clearance is the volume of plasma that supplies the excreted 20 mmol; it is this volume that is completely cleared of its phosphate. How much plasma has to be completely cleared of phosphate to supply the 20 mmol? We know from the data that the plasma phosphate concentration equals 1 mmol/L. Therefore, it would take

$$\frac{20 \text{ mmol/day}}{1 \text{ mmol/L}} = 20 \text{ L/day}$$

to supply the excreted phosphate. Clearance of a substance answers the question: How much plasma must be completely cleared to supply the excreted mass of that substance? Accordingly, $C_{PO_4} = 20$ L/day.

BASIC CLEARANCE FORMULA

It should be evident, therefore, that the basic clearance formula for any substance X is

$$C_X = \frac{\text{mass of } X \text{ excreted/time}}{P_X}$$

$$C_X = \frac{U_X V}{P_X}$$

where C_X = clearance of substance X
   U_X = urine concentration of X
   V = urine volume per time
   P_X = arterial plasma concentration of X

C_{In} is a measure of GFR simply because the volume of plasma completely cleared of inulin, i.e., the volume from which the excreted inulin comes, is equal to the volume of plasma filtered. C_{PO_4} must be less than C_{In} because much of the filtered phosphate is reabsorbed; therefore, less plasma was cleared of phosphate than of inulin.

Thus, the following generalization emerges: Whenever the clearance of a freely filterable substance is less than the inulin clearance, tubular reabsorption of that substance must have occurred. This is simply another way of stating that whenever the mass of substance excreted in the urine is less than the mass filtered during the same period of time, tubular reabsorption must have occurred.

The phrase "freely filterable" is essential in the above generalization. Protein serves as an excellent example. The clearance of protein in a normal person is virtually zero, obviously lower than the C_{In}. However, this does not prove that protein is reabsorbed. The major reason for the zero clearance is that the protein is not filtered. Accordingly, to compare inulin clearance to the clearance of any completely or partially protein-bound substance (calcium, for example), one must use the filterable plasma concentration of the substance rather than the total plasma concentration in the clearance formula.

Is the clearance of creatinine in humans higher or lower than that of inulin? The answer is higher. Like inulin, creatinine is freely filtered and not reabsorbed; therefore, a volume of plasma equal to that of the GFR (i.e., the C_{In}) is completely cleared of creatinine. But in addition, a small amount of creatinine is secreted. Therefore, some plasma in addition to that filtered is cleared of its creatinine by means of tubular secretion. The clearance formula is precisely the same as that for any other substance:

$$C_{Cr} = \frac{U_{Cr}V}{P_{Cr}}$$

Another generalization emerges: Whenever the clearance of a substance is greater than inulin clearance, tubular secretion of that substance must have occurred. Again, this is merely another way of stating that whenever the excreted mass exceeds the filtered mass, secretion must be occurring.

Another substance secreted by the proximal tubules is the organic anion **para-aminohippurate (PAH)**. PAH is also filtered at the glomerulus, and, when its plasma concentration is fairly low, virtually all the PAH that escapes filtration is secreted. Since PAH is not reabsorbed, the net effect is that all the plasma supplying the nephrons is completely cleared of PAH. If PAH were completely cleared from all the plasma flowing through the *entire* kidney, its clearance would measure the **total renal plasma flow (TRPF)**. However, about 10 to 15 percent of the total renal plasma flow supplies nonsecreting portions of the kidneys, such as peripelvic fat and the medulla, and this plasma cannot, therefore, lose its PAH by secretion. Accordingly the PAH clearance actually measures the so-called **effective renal plasma flow (ERPF)** and is approximately 85 to 90 percent of the total renal plasma flow. The clearance formula for PAH is, of course,

$$C_{PAH} = \frac{U_{PAH}V}{P_{PAH}} = ERPF$$

Once we have measured the ERPF,[2] we can calculate easily the **effective renal blood flow (ERBF)**:

[2] To reiterate, C_{PAH} measures ERPF, not TRPF, because some PAH escapes filtration and secretion. However, we can measure the amount that has escaped by measuring the concentration of PAH in the renal venous plasma. We can then calculate TRPF by using that value in the following equation:

$$TRPF = \frac{U_{PAH}V}{arterial_{PAH} - renal\ venous_{PAH}}$$

This equation is simply an example of the law of conservation of mass: What comes in at the renal artery must go out through the renal vein and urine combined.

$$ERBF = \frac{ERPF}{1 - V_c}$$

where V_c = the blood hematocrit, i.e., the fraction of blood occupied by erythrocytes

It should be emphasized that C_{PAH} measures ERPF only when plasma PAH is fairly low. If plasma PAH were increased to a level so high that the PAH secretory T_m were exceeded, PAH would not be completely removed from the plasma supplying the nephrons and the use of its clearance as a measure of ERPF would be invalid. Another substance that is handled in a manner similar to PAH is diodrast; accordingly, C_D is also a measure of ERPF.

Urea clearance C_{urea} can be determined by the usual formula:

$$C_{urea} = \frac{U_{urea}V}{P_{urea}}$$

Urea, like inulin, is freely filterable, but approximately 50 percent of filtered urea is reabsorbed; therefore, C_{urea} will be approximately 50 percent of C_{In}. If the mass of urea reabsorbed were always *exactly* 50 percent of that filtered, could C_{urea} be used to estimate GFR? The answer is yes. One would merely multiply the C_{urea} by 2 to obtain a value equal to the GFR. Unfortunately, as will be described in Chap. 4, urea reabsorption varies between 40 and 60 percent of the filtered urea, so that one cannot merely multiply by 2. Nonetheless, the urea clearance is easy to perform clinically and can be used as at least a crude indicator of GFR. The creatinine clearance is certainly a better way of evaluating GFR. But recall that because of creatinine secretion, it is not completely accurate either.

QUANTITATION OF TUBULAR REABSORPTION AND SECRETION USING CLEARANCE METHODS

To reiterate, once a method (determination of C_{In}) is available for measuring GFR, it becomes possible to determine whether the overall nephron manifests net reabsorption or net secretion of any given substance. If the clearance of the substance (using the filterable plasma concentration in the calculation) is less than that of inulin, net reabsorption must be occurring; if the clearance of the substance is greater than that of inulin, net secretion exists.

Why the word *net* in the above statements? The finding that a substance's clearance is less than that of inulin definitely proves reabsorption but does not disprove secretion; secretion might also have been present but masked by a greater rate of reabsorption. Similarly, proof of the presence of overall secretion ($C_X > C_{In}$) does not disprove the possibility that reabsorption, too, is present but of lesser magnitude than secretion.

Calculation of the magnitude of the *net* reabsorption or secretion in units of mass per time is given for any substance by the following equation:

$$\underset{(U_X V)}{\text{Mass excreted}} = \underset{\substack{(GFR \times P_X) \\ (C_{In} \times P_X)}}{\text{mass filtered}} + \text{mass secreted} - \text{mass reabsorbed}$$

Rearranging terms,

$$\underset{(C_{In} \times P_X)}{\text{Mass filtered}} - \underset{(U_X V)}{\text{mass excreted}} = (\text{mass reabsorbed} - \text{mass secreted})$$

Note that reabsorption and secretion are not *directly* measured variables but are derived as a single net value from the measurements of filtered and excreted masses. A positive value (filtered > excreted) quantifies net reabsorption, and a negative value (filtered < excreted) net secretion. (We have previously used this type of quantitation several times without formally defining it, for example, in Chap. 2, for the calculation of glucose T_m.)

Another common way of quantitating the degree of net reabsorption or net secretion is as **fractional excretion (FE)**. FE answers this question: What fraction of the filtered mass of a substance does the excreted mass represent?

$$\frac{\text{Mass excreted}}{\text{Mass filtered}} = \text{fractional excretion}$$

$$\frac{U_X V}{GFR \times P_x} = FE_X$$

Thus, for example, an FE_X of 0.23 means that, overall, the mass of X excreted is 23 percent of the mass of X filtered; therefore 77 percent of the filtered X has undergone net reabsorption. An FE_X of 1.5 means that

50 percent *more* X is excreted than was filtered; i.e., secretion is occurring.[3]

PLASMA CREATININE AND UREA CONCENTRATIONS AS INDICATORS OF GFR CHANGES

As described previously, the creatinine clearance is a close approximation of the GFR and is, therefore, a valuable clinical determination.

$$C_{Cr} = \frac{U_{Cr}V}{P_{Cr}}$$

In practice, however, it is far more common to measure plasma creatinine alone and to use this as an *indicator* of GFR. This approach is justified by the fact that most excreted creatinine gains entry to the tubule by filtration. If we ignore the small amount secreted, there should be an excellent

---

[3] Note that when inulin is used to measure GFR, the formula for fractional excretion is simply the ratio of C_X/C_{In}:

$$\frac{U_X V/P_X}{U_{In} V/P_{In}} = FE_X$$

Moreover, since urine volume (V) is common to both clearances, it is not even necessary to measure V to calculate a fractional excretion:

$$\frac{U_X/P_X}{U_{In}/P_{In}} = FE_X$$

An analogous double ratio is the key to evaluation, using micropuncture, not overall tubular function but the presence of net reabsorption or net secretion in individual nephron segments. Let us take the handling of the hypothetical substance Q by the proximal tubule as an example. A sample of fluid is collected from the end of the proximal tubule in an experimental animal given inulin, and its concentrations of Q and inulin are measured and compared to those of arterial plasma. The fraction of filtered Q remaining at the end of the proximal tubule is given by the ratio:

$$\frac{\text{Tubular fluid}_Q/\text{Plasma}_Q}{\text{Tubular fluid}_{In}/\text{Plasma}_{In}}$$

Let us assume that the value is found to be approximately 0.6; i.e., about 60 percent of the filtered Q remains at the end of the proximal tubule. This means that 40 percent of the filtered Q had been reabsorbed by the proximal tubule.

To determine what the loop of Henle has done, a sample of fluid is collected from the very early distal convoluted tubule and the "double ratio" for it is compared with that for the end of the proximal; it is found to be 1.1, compared to 0.6 for the late proximal, establishing that Q has been secreted into the loop. Similarly, a late distal convoluted sample can be compared with the early distal one to evaluate the net contribution of the distal convoluted tubule.

inverse correlation between plasma creatinine and GFR, as shown by the following example.

A normal person's plasma creatinine is 10 mg/L. It remains stable because each day the amount of creatinine produced is excreted. One day the GFR suddenly decreases permanently by 50 percent because of a blood clot in the renal artery. On that day the person filters only 50 percent as much creatinine as normal, so that creatinine excretion is also reduced by 50 percent. (We are ignoring the small contribution of secreted creatinine.) Therefore, assuming no change in creatinine production, the person goes into positive creatinine balance, and the plasma creatinine rises. But despite the persistent 50 percent GFR reduction, the plasma creatinine does not continue to rise indefinitely; rather, it stabilizes at 20 mg/L, i.e., after it has doubled. At this point the person once again is able to excrete creatinine at the normal rate and so remains stable. The reason is that the 50 percent GFR reduction has been counterbalanced by the doubling of plasma creatinine, and filtered creatinine is again normal.

$$\text{Original normal state: Filtered creatinine} = 10 \text{ mg/L} \times 180 \text{ L/day}$$
$$= 1800 \text{ mg/day}$$
$$\text{New steady state: Filtered creatinine} = 20 \text{ mg/L} \times 90 \text{ L/day}$$
$$= 1800 \text{ mg/day}$$

What if the GFR then fell to 30 L/day? Again creatinine retention would occur until a new steady state had been established, i.e., until the person is again filtering 1800 mg/day. What would the new plasma creatinine be?

$$1800 \text{ mg/day} = P_{Cr} \times 30 \text{ L/day}$$
$$P_{Cr} = 60 \text{ mg/L}$$

It should now be clear why a single plasma creatinine is a reasonable indicator of GFR (Fig. 3-1). It is not completely accurate, however, for three reasons: (1) Some creatinine is secreted. (2) There is no way of knowing exactly what the person's original creatinine was when GFR was normal. (3) Creatinine production may not remain completely unchanged.

Since urea is also handled by filtration, the same type of analysis would indicate that the measurement of plasma urea concentration could serve as an indicator of GFR. However, it is a much less accurate indicator than plasma creatinine because the range of normal plasma urea concentration varies widely, depending on protein intake and changes in tissue catabolism, and because urea is reabsorbed to a *variable* degree.

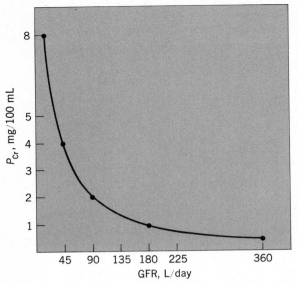

Figure 3-1 Steady-state relationship between GFR and plasma creatinine, assuming no creatinine is secreted.

(The fact that it is reabsorbed would not interfere with its use as an indicator if the reabsorption were always a *fixed* percentage of the filtered mass.)

Study questions: 13 to 23

4

RENAL HANDLING
OF ORGANIC SUBSTANCES

OBJECTIVES

The student understands the renal handling of certain organic substances.

1 States the major characteristics of the proximal-tubular systems for reabsorption of organic nutrients
2 Describes the renal handling of proteins and linear peptides
3 Describes the renal handling of urea
4 Describes the proximal secretory system for organic anions; describes the overall renal handling of PAH
5 Describes the renal handling of urate
6 Describes the proximal secretory system for organic cations
7 Describes, in general terms, the renal handling of weak acids and bases, including the contributions of glomerular filtration, active proximal secretion, and passive movements secondary to water reabsorption or pH changes; given any change in luminal pH, predicts the change in net transtubular movement for a substance with a particular pK

Subsequent chapters of this book will deal almost exclusively with the renal handling of inorganic substances since regulation of their excretion constitutes the kidneys' major physiological role. However, as pointed out in Chap. 1, another major renal function is the excretion of organic waste products, foreign chemicals, and their metabolites. Moreover, reabsorptive processes must exist to prevent massive excretion of filtered organic nutrients. An analysis of the renal transport pathways for all these organic substances is well beyond the scope of this book, but this chapter briefly describes certain of the major ones.

GLUCOSE, AMINO ACIDS, ET AL.:
PROXIMAL REABSORPTION OF ORGANIC NUTRIENTS

The proximal tubule is the major site for reabsorption of the large quantities of organic nutrients filtered each day by the renal corpuscles. These include glucose, amino acids, several Krebs cycle intermediates, certain water-soluble vitamins, lactate, acetoacetate, β-hydroxybutyrate, and still others. The characteristics of glucose reabsorption described in examples used earlier in Chap. 2 are typical of the transport processes for most (but not all) of them:

1 They are active in that they can reabsorb their respective solutes against electrochemical gradients. Indeed the intraluminal concentration of the substance can often be reduced virtually to zero. Such marked transtubular concentration gradients can be established for these organic nutrients because there is only a modest "leak" of the molecules from the interstital fluid back into the lumen across the tight junctions between cells. The statement made in a previous chapter that the proximal tubule is "leaky" and, hence, unable to achieve large concentration gradients concerned inorganic ions, not organic solutes.

2 The "uphill" step is across the luminal membrane, usually via cotransport with sodium. Movement across the basolateral membrane from cell into interstitium is by facilitated diffusion.[1]

3 They manifest T_ms that are usually well above the amounts *normally* filtered. Accordingly, the kidneys protect against loss of the substances but do not help set their plasma concentrations. However, as we saw for glucose in diabetic persons, the plasma concentration of any of these substances may become so increased under abnormal conditions that it causes the reabsorptive T_m for it to be exceeded and large quantities to be lost in the urine. Good examples are acetocetate and β-hydroxybutyrate in patients with severe uncontrolled diabetes.

4 They manifest specificity. This statement means that there are a large number of different carriers, i.e., membrane proteins with which the different solute types interact. But there is by no means a one-to-one correspondence since two or more closely related substances may utilize the same carrier. For example, the amino acid reabsorptive mechanisms are quite distinct from those for glucose and other monosaccharides, but there are not 20 separate processes, one for each amino acid. Rather there is one for arginine, lysine, and ornithine; another for glutamate and aspartate; and so on. Shared pathways allow competition among those substances utilizing any given pathway. For example, the administration of large quantities of ornithine partially blocks the reabsorption of the other amino acids that share its pathway. This is, of course, explainable on the basis of competition for the common carrier's binding sites.

5 They are inhibitable by a variety of drugs and diseases. There are persons with genetic defects manifested as a deficit in one or more of these proximal reabsorptive systems. In some cases, the deficit may be

---

[1] For discussion of the mechanism of movement across the basolateral membrane, see Guggino and Guggino, and Zelikovic and Chesney, in Suggested Readings. Also, for some amino acids, "uphill" transport from interstitial fluid into cell, i.e., in the direction opposite the reabsorptive movement, has been demonstrated. Presence of this basolateral carrier explains why, under certain circumstances, net secretion, rather than net reabsorption, of these amino acids occurs. The physiological significance of these carriers is that they supply amino acids for the cell's own metabolic requirements. (See Schafer and Williams, and Silbernagel, in Suggested Readings.)

highly specific (e.g., involving only one amino acid), whereas in others, multiple systems may be involved (e.g., glucose and many amino acids). This range of defects is also seen when the deficit is due to an external agent (e.g., lead toxicity) rather than to a genetic abnormality.

PROTEINS AND PEPTIDES

The proximal tubule is also the major site for protein reabsorption, and it is listed separately here to emphasize its importance and the fact that its reabsorptive pathway is quite different from those for the substances described in the preceding section. Indeed, as we shall see, the term *reabsorption*, though widely used, is really a misnomer.

As mentioned, there is a very small amount of protein in the glomerular filtrate. The normal concentration approximates 10 mg/L, about 0.02 percent of plasma albumin concentration (50 g/L). Yet because of the huge volume of fluid filtered per day, this concentration is not negligible.

$$\begin{aligned} \text{Total filtered protein} &= \text{GFR} \times \text{filtrate conc of protein} \\ &= 180 \text{ L/day} \times 10 \text{ mg/L} \\ &= 1.8 \text{ g/day} \end{aligned}$$

If none of this protein were reabsorbed, the entire 1.8 g would be lost in the urine. In fact, virtually all the filtered protein is reabsorbed, so that the excretion of protein in the urine is normally only 100 mg/day. The mechanism by which protein is reabsorbed is easily saturated, so any large increase in filtered protein resulting from increased glomerular permeability can cause the excretion of large quantities of protein. For example, suppose that disease causes the renal corpuscles to allow 1 percent of the plasma albumin to be filtered:

$$\begin{aligned} \text{Filtered albumin} &= \text{GFR} \times (50 \text{ g/L}) (0.01) \\ &= 180 \text{ L/day} \times 0.5 \text{ g/L} \\ &= 90 \text{ g/day} \end{aligned}$$

This is far greater than the reabsorptive T_m for protein, and huge quantities of albumin would be lost in the urine.

The initial step in protein reabsorption is endocytosis at the luminal membrane. This energy-requiring process is triggered by the binding of filtered protein molecules to specific sites on the luminal membrane. Therefore, the rate of endocytosis is increased in proportion to the concentration of protein in the glomerular filtrate until a maximal rate of vesicle formation, and thus the T_m for protein reabsorption, is reached.

The pinched-off intracellular vesicles resulting from endocytosis merge with lysosomes, whose enzymes degrade the protein to low-molecular-weight fragments, mainly individual amino acids. These end products then exit the cells across the basolateral membrane into the interstitial fluid, from which they gain entry to the peritubular capillaries.

It should be evident from this description that the term *reabsorption*, in reference to protein handling, is not really accurate since the intact protein molecules themselves are not actually being moved from lumen to interstitial fluid but are catabolized in the renal-tubular cells. Nevertheless, the important point is that the filtered protein is not excreted in the urine and is, in this sense, reabsorbed. There may be a small number of intact molecules that actually do make the trip since a few intact endocytotic vesicles move through the cell cytoplasm and empty their proteins by exocytosis into the interstitial fluid.

Discussions of the renal handling of protein logically tend to focus on albumin since it is by far the most abundant plasma protein. There are, of course, many other plasma proteins, and it should be emphasized here that many of these proteins, being smaller than albumin, are filtered to a greater degree than albumin. For example, growth hormone (m.w. = 20,000) is approximately 60 percent filterable. This means that relatively large fractions of these smaller plasma proteins are filtered and then degraded in tubular cells. Accordingly, the kidneys are major sites of catabolism of many plasma proteins, including polypeptide hormones, and decreased rates of degradation occurring in renal disease may result in elevated plasma hormone concentrations.

Smaller linear polypeptides, such as angiotensin II, are handled quite differently than proteins. They are completely filterable at the renal corpuscles and are then catabolized, mainly into amino acids, within the proximal tubular lumen by peptidases located on the luminal plasma membrane. The amino acids, as well as di-and tripeptides either generated by this process or filtered, are then reabsorbed.

Finally, it should be noted that in certain types of renal damage, proteins released from tubular cells rather than filtered at the renal corpuscles may appear in the urine and provide important diagnostic information.

UREA

Just as glucose provides an excellent example of an actively reabsorbed solute, urea, the primary end product of protein catabolism, provides an example of reabsorption by diffusion. Urea is a highly diffusible substance, so that net movement across most biological membranes requires only the creation of a diffusion gradient for it. Such gradients exist within the kidneys, as the following analysis shows.

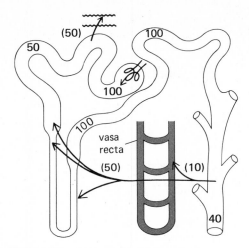

Figure 4-1 Major pathways for the renal handling of urea. The numbers in the tubule denote the percentages of filtered urea at various sites along the tubule. It is not clear whether most of the secreted urea enters the straight portions of the proximal tubules or the thin limbs of Henle's loop. Not shown in the figure is the fact that a very small amount of urea is reabsorbed by the distal convoluted tubules and cortical collecting ducts. *(Redrawn from H Valtin, Renal Function: Mechanisms Preserving Fluid and Solute Balance in Health, Boston, Little, Brown, 1973.)*

Since urea is freely filtered at the renal corpuscle, its concentration in Bowman's capsule is identical to its concentration in peritubular-capillary plasma. Then, as the fluid flows along the proximal convoluted tubule, water reabsorption occurs, increasing the concentration of any intra-tubular solute not being reabsorbed at the same rate as the water. As a result, the concentration of urea in the tubular lumen becomes greater than the concentration of urea in the peritubular plasma. Accordingly, urea is able to diffuse down this concentration gradient from tubular lumen to interstitial fluid and then into peritubular capillaries. Urea reab-sorption is, thus, a passive process and completely dependent on water reabsorption, which establishes the diffusion gradient.

Beyond the proximal convoluted tubule, the story becomes much more complicated. Let us pick up the fluid at the end of the proximal convoluted tubule, by which point approximately 50 percent of the urea has been reabsorbed as just described, and follow it the rest of the way, using Fig. 4-1 as reference.

What happens in the straight portion of the proximal tubule and Henle's loop? You might logically have predicted that more urea would be reabsorbed along with the water reabsorbed from these nephron seg-ments, but such turns out not to be the case. By the beginning of the distal convoluted tubule, there is actually twice as much urea in the tubular fluid as originally left the proximal convoluted tubule, i.e., about the same amount as originally filtered! Thus, for the straight proximal tubule and

Henle's loop, taken together, net *secretion* of urea has occurred. This secretion is mainly into the proximal straight tubule and thin limb of Henle's loop. The thick ascending limb does not secrete urea.[2]

However, the source of this secreted urea is *not* peritubular plasma, the usual source of secreted solutes, and is best ignored for the present until we complete the tubular fluid's journey through the nephron.

Very little of the large amount of urea reaching the distal convoluted tubule is reabsorbed there or in the next segment, the cortical collecting duct, because these two tubular segments are relatively impermeable to urea. Therefore, most of the urea in the fluid that entered the distal convoluted tubule from the loop will reach the medullary collecting ducts. There, particularly in the inner medulla, passive urea reabsorption once again becomes quite large both because of a high tubular permeability to urea and because of the extensive water reabsorption there. The urea that escapes reabsorption by the medullary collecting ducts amounts to approximately 40 percent of the amount originally filtered, and this is the urea excreted into the final urine. Thus, the *overall* net renal-tubular handling of urea along the entire nephron is the reabsorption of approximately 60 percent.

Now we can back up and point out the source of the urea that entered the proximal straight tubule and the thin loop of Henle by secretion—it is urea that was reabsorbed by the medullary collecting ducts. As illustrated in Fig. 4-1, as the urea diffuses out of the medullary collecting ducts into the interstitial fluid, the urea concentration of this fluid is raised, thereby creating a gradient for net diffusion of urea into the straight proximal tubule and thin loops of Henle.

Thus, most of the urea that diffuses *out of* the medullary collecting ducts (reabsorption) diffuses *into* the proximal straight tubules and thin loops (secretion) and once more flows through the distal convoluted tubules and cortical collecting ducts, only to suffer the same fate in the medullary collecting ducts. In other words, a large quantity of urea is simply recycled along the tubule. Not all the urea that diffuses out of the medullary collecting ducts is recycled in this manner, however, since some enters the medullary capillaries and is carried out of the kidneys.

In summary, the renal handling of filtered urea is by diffusion.[3] Approximately 50 percent is reabsorbed into the blood across the proximal convoluted tubule. The remaining 50 percent undergoes a recycling sequence beyond the proximal convoluted tubule characterized by reabsorption out of the medullary collecting ducts, followed by secretion into the proximal straight tubules and thin loops of Henle. Some urea escapes

[2] Indeed, it probably reabsorbs urea (see Knepper and Roch-Ramel in Suggested Readings).

[3] It is possible that some component of *active* reabsorption and/or secretion also exists along with these dominant passive components (see Knepper and Roch-Ramel in Suggested Readings).

this recycling and makes it into the medullary capillaries and back into the systemic circulation. The net result is that approximately 60 percent (50 percent by the proximal and 10 percent by the rest of the nephron) of the filtered urea is truly (in the sense of "irrevocably") reabsorbed.

This figure of 60 percent reabsorbed applies to situations in which the urine flow is relatively low, i.e., water reabsorption is high. Only about 40 percent of the filtered urea is reabsorbed when the urine flow is high, i.e., water reabsorption is low. This occurs because the diffusion gradient for urea reabsorption is created by water reabsorption, and so when water reabsorption is low, a smaller urea gradient will be created.

To reiterate, the net reabsorption of filtered urea ranges between 40 and 60 percent. A crucial fact is that this same range applies regardless of how high the plasma urea concentration may be. Thus, urea reabsorption manifests no true T_m in absolute terms because it is governed by diffusion gradients and requires no interaction with membrane binding sites.

PAH, URATE, ET AL.: PROXIMAL SECRETION OF ORGANIC ANIONS

The proximal tubule actively secretes a large number of different organic anions, both foreign and endogenously produced (see Table 4-1 for a partial listing). Many of the organic anions handled by this system are also filterable at the renal corpuscles, and so the amount secreted proximally adds to that which gains entry to the tubule via glomerular filtration. Others, however, are extensively bound to plasma proteins and so undergo glomerular filtration only to a limited extent; accordingly, proximal-tubular secretion constitutes the only significant mechanism for their excretion (recall from Chap. 2 that binding to plasma proteins does not generally impede tubular secretion).

Table 4-1 Some Organic Anions
Actively Secreted by the Proximal Tubule

Endogenous Substances	Drugs
Bile salts	Acetazolamide
Fatty acids	Chlorothiazide
Hippurates	Ethacrynate
Hydroxybenzoates	Furosemide
Oxalate	Penicillin
Prostaglandins	Probenecid
Urate	Saccharin
	Salicylates
	Sulfonamides

The active secretory pathway for organic anions in the proximal tubule has a relatively low specificity; i.e., a single system (or possibly several very closely related ones) is responsible for the secretion of all the organic anions listed in Table 4-1 and many more. The relatively non-discriminating nature of this system accounts for its ability to eliminate from the body so many drugs and other foreign environmental chemicals. In this regard the liver's metabolic transformations are frequently important; in the liver, many foreign (and endogenous) substances are conjugated with either glucuronate or sulfate, and these two types of conjugates are actively transported by the organic-anion secretory pathway.

The most intensively studied organic anion secreted by this pathway is **para-aminohippurate (PAH)**, the substance, as we saw in Chap. 3, that is used for the measurement of effective renal plasma flow. PAH is actively transported into proximal tubular cells across the basolateral membrane, and the resulting high intracellular concentration then provides the gradient for the facilitated diffusion of PAH across the luminal membrane into the tubular lumen.[4]

This mechanism for PAH secretion is shared by the other organic anions secreted proximally; i.e., they all share the same carriers. As might be predicted, there is competition for transport among these anions, so that an elevated plasma concentration of one of the substances will tend to inhibit the secretion of the others. Thus, drugs used deliberately to inhibit proximal organic-anion secretion are usually, themselves, organic anions.

Another characteristic of this secretory system is T_m limitation: As the plasma concentration of an anion secreted by the system increases, so does the rate of secretion until the T_m for that substance is reached, beyond which no further increase in secretion occurs. This direct relationship between plasma concentration and rate of secretion, at values below T_m, provides a simple but effective mechanism for homeostatically regulating the endogenous organic anions handled by the system and for speeding the excretion of foreign anions.

PAH is typical, in yet another way, of many (but not all) of the organic anions secreted proximally: It undergoes no significant tubular reabsorption anywhere along the nephron. Accordingly, the mass of PAH excreted per unit time is equal to the sum of the mass filtered—PAH is not protein-bound—and the mass secreted.

In contrast, some of the other organic anions secreted proximally can undergo significant passive tubular reabsorption, mainly in more distal nephron segments, and the mechanisms of this passive reabsorption will be described in the last section of this chapter.

Finally, there are a few proximally secreted organic anions that also undergo *active* tubular reabsorption, in most cases also in the proximal tubule. The most notable example is urate. The major form of uric acid in

[4] The basolateral entry step is a secondary active process—cotransport or countertransport with an inorganic ion (see Moller and Sheikh in Suggested Readings).

plasma is ionized urate. Urate is not protein-bound and so is freely filterable at the renal corpuscles. Urate undergoes, mainly in the proximal tubule, both active tubular reabsorption and active tubular secretion. The rate of tubular reabsorption is normally much greater than the rate of tubular secretion, and so the net tubular effect is to remove urate from the lumen. This occurrence explains why, in normal persons, the mass of urate excreted per unit time is only a small fraction of the mass filtered. Although urate reabsorption is more extensive than secretion, it seems to be the rate of the secretory process that is homeostatically controlled to maintain relative constancy of plasma urate. In other words, if plasma urate begins to increase because of increased urate production, the rate of active proximal secretion of urate is stimulated, thereby increasing urate excretion.

Many persons have elevated plasma concentrations of urate because they secrete and, hence, excrete less of this substance at any given plasma urate concentration than do normal persons. Two other causes of kidney-caused elevations of plasma urate are: (1) decreased filtration of urate secondary to decreased GFR and (2) excessive reabsorption of urate.

PROXIMAL SECRETION OF ORGANIC CATIONS

Proximal tubules possess an active transport system (or several closely related systems) for organic cations that is analogous to that for organic anions. It is relatively nonspecific in that it transports a large number of foreign and endogenously occurring substances (Table 4-2) that compete with each other for transport, and it manifests a T_m limitation.

The proximal secretion of organic anions, just as the proximal secretion of organic cations, is particularly critical for the excretion of those substances extensively bound to plasma proteins and not filterable at the renal corpuscle. However, again similar to the case for the organic

Table 4-2   Some Organic Cations Actively Secreted by the Proximal Tubule

Endogenous Substances	Drugs
Acetylcholine	Atropine
Choline	Isoproterenol
Creatinine	Cimetidine
Dopamine	Meperidine
Epinephrine	Morphine
Guanidine	Procaine
Histamine	Quinine
Serotonin	Tetraethyl ammonium
Norepinephrine	
Thiamine	

anions, many of the organic cations secreted by the proximal tubules are not protein-bound and therefore also undergo glomerular filtration as well as tubular secretion; creatinine is a good example.

Finally, and again analogous to the story for organic anions, some organic cations are not only actively secreted by the proximal tubules but may also undergo other forms of tubular handling, mainly passive reabsorption or secretion, a subject to which we now turn.

PASSIVE REABSORPTION OR SECRETION OF WEAK ORGANIC ACIDS AND BASES

Many organic anions and cations are the ionized forms, respectively, of weak acids and bases. Quite apart from any active tubular handling—mainly the proximal secretion described above—such substances, in their nonionized forms, may also undergo passive reabsorption or passive secretion, depending on several conditions, the most important being the pH of the urine. To be specific, many weak acids undergo net passive tubular secretion when the urine is highly alkaline but net passive tubular reabsorption when it is acidic. The opposite pattern is seen for many weak organic bases.

To understand what accounts for this pH dependency, one must realize that the renal-tubular epithelium, like other biological membranes, is mainly a lipid barrier. Accordingly, highly lipid-soluble substances can penetrate it fairly readily by diffusion. Recall that one of the major determinants of lipid solubility is the polarity of a molecule; the more polar, the less lipid-soluble. Now, a weak acid exists as a polar ion in alkaline solution and as a nonpolar molecule in acid solution:

$$A^- + H^+ \rightleftharpoons AH$$

In contrast, for weak bases, the ionic form is favored in acid solutions:

$$B + H^+ \rightleftharpoons BH^+$$

Accordingly, the diffusible form of weak acids is generated in acidic fluid, whereas the diffusible form of weak bases is generated in alkaline fluid.

Let us now apply these principles, using aspirin as an example and ignoring, for the moment, active proximal secretion of aspirin:

$$\underset{\text{(acetylsalicylate)}}{ASA^-} + H^+ \rightleftharpoons \underset{\text{(acetylsalicylic acid)}}{ASA\text{-}H}$$

Aspirin is filterable at the renal corpuscles, and so its concentration in Bowman's space is identical to that in peritubular plasma. Moreover,

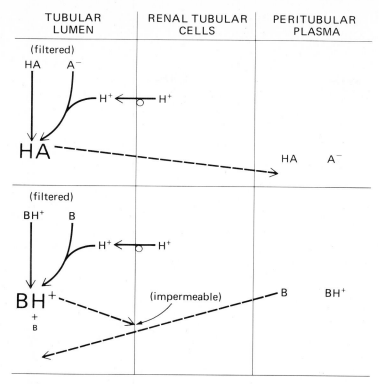

TUBULAR LUMEN	RENAL TUBULAR CELLS	PERITUBULAR PLASMA

Figure 4-2 Acidification of the luminal fluid creates, by mass action, the gradients that drive net passive reabsorption (→) of weak acids (top) and net passive secretion (←) of weak bases (bottom).

because the pH of the glomerular filtrate is identical to that of peritubular plasma, the relative proportions of ASA$^-$ and ASH-H are also the same in the two fluids. As the filtered fluid flows along the tubule, water is reabsorbed, and this removal of solvent concentrates both ASA$^-$ and ASA-H, thereby creating lumen-to-plasma diffusion gradients favoring net reabsorption (exactly as described for urea). However, since only ASA-H can penetrate the membrane to any great extent, only this form is reabsorbed. Simultaneously, and this is really the crucial point, secretion of hydrogen ions into the lumen lowers the luminal pH and favors, by mass action, the generation of ASA-H, which can then diffuse along its concentration gradient from lumen to peritubular plasma (Fig. 4-2). In other words, water reabsorption is one factor that helps create the concentration gradient required for passive reabsorption, but luminal acidification, by generating the diffusible form of the substance from the nondiffusible form, is even more important in creating the gradient.

The story is even more interesting, however, for as we shall see in Chap. 9, the tubular fluid can be made alkaline rather than more acid under certain circumstances. This would shift the intraluminal reaction toward generation of ASA$^-$ at the expense of ASA-H, and the resulting decrease in luminal ASA-H would, of course, reduce the gradient for net reabsorption. Indeed, luminal ASA-H might actually fall below peritubular-capillary plasma ASA-H, thereby establishing a gradient for net passive *secretion* of ASA-H rather than reabsorption. Thus, the net passive reabsorption of weak organic acids is inversely related to urine pH, and net passive secretion may be seen when the urine is alkaline.

We have been dealing only qualitatively with these concepts. The quantitative relationship is determined by the pK of the acid and the pH of the tubular fluid. For example, an acid with a pK well below the lowest tubular-fluid pH achievable—4.4—would always exist within the tubule almost entirely in the anionic (nondiffusible) form and thus always undergo relatively little passive reabsorption. In contrast, an organic acid with a pK of 6 would exhibit a marked increase in the degree of passive reabsorption if intratubular-fluid pH were lowered from 7 to 5 since the nonionized (diffusible) form would go from 10 percent of the total to 90 percent. Because pH changes are, as we shall see, greatest in the more distal tubular segments, these segments are the major sites for such pH-dependent passive transport.

Let us apply these same concepts to the passive renal-tubular handling of weak bases: When the tubular fluid is highly acidic, the generation of BH$^+$ from B is favored. The BH$^+$ cannot diffuse out of the lumen because of its charge, but the lowering of intraluminal B favors net passive secretion of B from peritubular-capillary plasma into the lumen. Conversely, when the urine is alkaline, generation of B within the lumen is favored, and a gradient is established for net passive reabsorption. Thus, weak bases are reabsorbed passively when the urine is alkaline but may be passively secreted when it is acid.

It must be reemphasized that the description in this section has been in terms of only *passive* reabsorption and secretion of these substances. The fact is, as described earlier in this chapter, *active* secretory mechanisms also exist in the proximal tubule for the anionic and cationic forms of many weak acids and bases. Accordingly, these forms may be actively secreted into the proximal-tubular lumen, followed by either passive reabsorption or passive secretion of the nonionized forms there and in the subsequent nephron segments, depending in part on urine flow rate but mainly on the change in luminal pH occurring along the tubule.

In summary, the excretion of a weak acid or base reflects the following factors:

1 The amount filtered at the renal corpuscle; this is determined by the product of the GFR and the ultrafilterable (non-protein-bound) plasma concentration of the substance.

2 The amount secreted actively by the proximal tubules; this increases with increasing plasma concentration until the T_m for that substance is reached. It is also sensitive to inhibition by competing anions.

3 The amount passively reabsorbed or secreted; this reflects the urine flow rate, the pK of the substance, and the pH of the urine.

Because so many medically used drugs are weak organic acids and bases, all these factors have important clinical implications. For example, if one wished to enhance the excretion of a drug that is a weak acid, one would attempt to alkalinize the urine. In contrast, acidification of the urine is desirable if one wished to prevent excretion of the drug. Of course, exactly the opposite would apply to weak organic bases. Increasing the urine flow would increase the excretion of both weak acids and bases. Finally, excretion could be reduced by giving another drug that interferes with any active proximal secretory pathway for the drug.

Study questions: 24 to 27

5

CONTROL OF RENAL HEMODYNAMICS

OBJECTIVES

The student understands the control of renal hemodynamics.

1   States the formula relating flow, pressure, and resistance
2   Knows the normal rates of GFR, RPF, and RBF; defines filtration fraction
3   Defines autoregulation of RBF and GFR; states the condition in which "pure" autoregulation can be observed; states the adaptive function of autoregulation
4   Describes the myogenic and tubuloglomerular feedback concepts to explain autoregulation
5   States how tubuloglomerular feedback lowers GFR when proximal reabsorption is inhibited
6   Describes the role of the renal sympathetic nerves and states the reflexes that cause their activity to increase
7   Describes how increases in renal sympathetic nerve activity cause filtration fraction to increase
8   States the effect of angiotensin II on renal arterioles and glomerular mesangial cells
9   Describes the four major controls of renin secretion; identifies the type of adrenergic receptor involved in the direct sympathetic pathway
10 States the adaptive value of the renal vasoconstriction induced by the renal nerves and angiotensin II
11 States the effect of the renal nerves and angiotensin II on renal prostaglandin synthesis and the function served by the prostaglandins
12 States the effect of antidiuretic hormone on renal arterioles
13 States the distribution of blood flow between cortex and medulla

The blood flow to the kidneys—the **RBF**—in a typical adult is approximately 1.1 L/min. Thus, the kidneys receive 20 to 25 percent of the total cardiac output (5L/min) even though their combined weight is less than 1 percent of total-body weight. Given a normal hematocrit of 0.45, the **total renal plasma flow (TRPF)** = 0.55 × 1.1 L/min = 605 mL/min. Recall that the GFR equals 125 mL/min. Therefore, of the 605 mL of plasma that enters the glomeruli via the afferent arterioles, 125/605, or 20 percent,

68

filters into Bowman's capsule, the remaining 480 mL passing via the efferent arterioles into the peritubular capillaries. This ratio—GFR/ TRPF—is known as the **filtration fraction.**

The basic equation for blood flow through any organ is

Organ blood flow = ∆P/R

where ∆ P = mean arterial pressure minus venous pressure for that organ
R = resistance to flow through that organ

Normally, the major determinant of resistance is the radii of the arterioles within that organ, itself determined mainly by the degree of contraction of the smooth muscle. It should be evident, therefore, that RBF is determined mainly by the mean arterial pressure and the contractile state of the renal arteriolar smooth muscle.

MEAN ARTERIAL PRESSURE AND AUTOREGULATION

Look again at the basic equation above. This equation predicts that if the pressure gradient is increased by 50 percent, blood flow will increase 50 percent. In the kidney, however, this prediction does not occur because the renal circulation manifests quite markedly the phenomenon of **autoregulation:** The RBF is relatively constant in the face of changes in mean renal arterial pressure when this pressure is changed over the range between 80 and 180 mmHg (Fig. 5-1).

If one isolates a kidney experimentally and perfuses it with blood by means of a pump, one can demonstrate that a 50 percent increase in renal arterial pressure produces less than a 10 percent increase in RBF. As seen in the above equation, there is only one possible explanation: Resistance in the kidney does not stay constant as arterial pressure increases. Rather, resistance automatically increases. The smooth muscle of the renal arterioles contracts to a greater degree, thereby decreasing the radii of the arterioles and, hence, increasing arteriolar resistance. Therefore, RBF remains relatively unchanged despite the increased arterial pressure.

This entire discussion applies not only to RBF but also to GFR, which also shows only small changes in the face of large changes in arterial pressure. There are several reasons for the fact that GFR, as well as RBF, is autoregulated. The most important is that the *afferent* arterioles are the major site of autoregulatory resistance changes in the face of arterial pressure changes. Accordingly, glomerular-capillary pressure and, therefore, net filtration pressure remain relatively unchanged. For example, a rise in renal arterial pressure triggers enhanced afferent-arteriolar constriction, thereby increasing the pressure drop between the

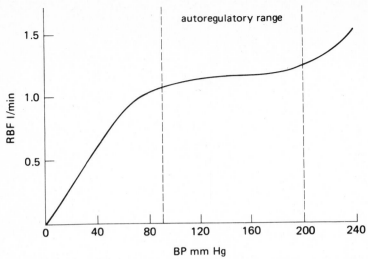

Figure 5-1   Autoregulation of renal blood flow (RBF). A similar pattern holds for glomerular filtration rate.

arteries and glomerular capillaries and preventing the transmission of the increased arterial pressure to the glomerular capillaries.

What is the mechanism of autoregulation; i.e., how does an increase in renal arterial pressure elicit enhanced contraction of the smooth muscle of renal arterioles, whereas a reduction in pressure elicits relaxation? One thing is for certain—the mechanism is completely intrarenal since it can be elicited in an isolated kidney perfused in vitro. Two intrarenal mechanisms are presently thought to be responsible for autoregulation: (1) **myogenic mechanism** and (2) **tubuloglomerular feedback.**

The myogenic mechanism is similar to that found in other (nonrenal) autoregulating vascular beds: Vascular smooth muscle contracts in response to increased stretch. Accordingly, an increased intra-arteriolar pressure distends the arteriolar wall, i.e., increases its passive tension, and the inherent response of the smooth muscle in the wall is to contract, thereby increasing the resistance offered by the vessel.

Tubuloglomerular feedback is a more complex process, which regulates GFR primarily, with changes in RBF being a secondary consequence. The basic pathway is illustrated in Fig. 5-2. Increased arterial pressure tends to raise both glomerular-capillary pressure (P_{GC}) and RBF. The increase in P_{GC} raises GFR and, hence, the rate of fluid flow through the proximal tubule and loop of Henle, including the macula densa. The macula densa cells somehow detect the increased flow past them, and this triggers the generation of a vasoconstrictor chemical by one of the cell types in the juxtaglomerular apparatus (JGA). This vasoconstrictor acts on the smooth muscle of the adjacent arterioles, particu-

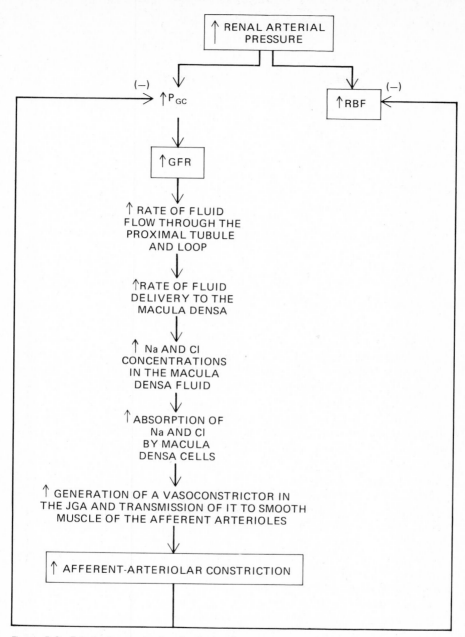

Figure 5-2 Tubuloglomerular feedback contribution to autoregulation.

larly the afferent arterioles, and causes vasoconstriction. The result is an increased afferent-arteriolar resistance, which decreases P_{GC} and, hence, GFR,[1] as well as RBF. Thus, this constriction counteracts the increases caused by the elevated renal arterial pressure.

A great deal remains unknown about tubuloglomerular feedback. First, how does the macula densa detect changes in rate of fluid flow? The most likely hypothesis at present is as follows (Fig. 5-2): When fluid delivery to the macula densa is increased, the fluid has increased sodium and chloride concentrations; this causes increased sodium and chloride reabsorption by the macula densa cells, and it is this increased reabsorption that generates the unknown immediate signal for increased vasoconstrictor production. A second unanswered question is the identity of the vasoconstrictor. Angiotensin II and prostaglandins may play permissive roles but are not the primary vasoconstrictors in tubuloglomerular feedback. **Adenosine,** which constricts renal arterioles, in contrast to its vasodilator effect on most other vascular beds, is a possibility, but conclusive evidence is still lacking.

The examples used to illustrate the myogenic and tubuloglomerular mechanisms used *increases* in renal arterial pressures as the initial event. It should be clear, however, that since mean arterial pressure is normally above the lower limit of the autoregulatory range (80 to 180 mmHg), *decreases* in arterial pressure will also be offset by the autoregulatory mechanisms: Decreased stretch of afferent-arteriolar smooth muscle causes relaxation, i.e., less contraction, and decreased flow through the macula densa causes less of the relevant vasoconstrictor to be produced by the JGA.

What is the adaptive value of autoregulation? First, as in any other autoregulating organ, it helps prevent major blood-flow changes in the face of arterial-pressure fluctuations. But it also serves a second role in the kidney, namely, the blunting of the large changes in solute and water excretion that would otherwise occur because of large changes in GFR whenever arterial pressure changed. This is the adaptive value of GFR autoregulation. Recall that the normal net filtration pressure in the glomeruli is only about 17mmHg. Accordingly, even relatively minor changes in arterial pressure could cause marked changes in glomerular-capillary pressure, GFR, and solute and water excretion, were the changes not effectively blunted by automatically elicited changes in afferent-arteriolar tonus.

In this regard, it should be emphasized that although we introduced tubuloglomerular feedback in the context of autoregulation, this pathway

---

[1] A decrease in P_{GC} may not be the only reason that GFR decreases. Some evidence suggests that the vasoconstrictor released by the JGA acts not only on the afferent arteriole but on the glomerular mesangial cells as well. As described earlier, contraction of these mesangial cells would reduce the surface area of the glomeruli, thereby decreasing the filtration coefficient (K_f) (see Briggs and Schnermann in Suggested Readings).

may also be important in situations characterized not by changes in arterial pressure but rather by disease-induced or drug-induced blockade of fluid reabsorption in the proximal tubule.[2] Under such conditions, the resulting increase in macula densa flow will trigger, via the usual sequence of events, a decrease in GFR and thereby limit the urinary loss of salt and water resulting from the defect in reabsorption. Note that in these cases, tubuloglomerular feedback actually causes GFR to go *down*, whereas during autoregulatory responses, it keeps GFR from changing.

Having pointed out the value of autoregulation, we must now emphasize three facts: (1) Autoregulation is not perfect; RBF and GFR *do change* when renal arterial pressure is changed, but they change to a much smaller degree than they would if autoregulation did not exist. (2) Autoregulation is virtually absent at mean arterial pressures below 70 mmHg and, therefore, cannot blunt GRF and RBF changes below this point. (3) Despite autoregulation, RBF and GFR can be altered considerably, even when the arterial pressure is within the autoregulatory range, by the factors to be described next—the sympathetic nervous system, the renin-angiotensin system, and prostaglandins.

SYMPATHETIC CONTROL

The afferent and efferent arterioles are richly supplied with sympathetic neurons, which cause, via alpha$_1$-adrenergic receptors, arteriolar constriction. Circulating **epinephrine** also activates these receptors.[3] In a resting, unstressed person, there is relatively little sympathetic tone to the kidneys, but a reflexly induced increase in sympathetic outflow will cause renal arteriolar constriction.

Because of this fact, in the above discussion of autoregulation, we set up artificial experimental conditions in which renal blood pressure was changed without altering blood pressure in the other arteries of the body; an analogue of this in a person might be an obstruction in a renal artery. Such experimental conditions are necessary to demonstrate autoregulation clearly because when the systemic arterial pressure decreases in the *intact* organism, neuroendocrine reflexes are brought into play that may mask the occurrence of autoregulation.

One of these responses is increased activity in the renal sympathetic nerves (and increased circulating epinephrine) reflexly mediated via the

[2] You might logically conclude that drugs that block loop fluid reabsorption would trigger tubuloglomerular feedback effects similar to those occuring with proximal-tubular blockade. However, loop-acting drugs block sodium and chloride reabsorption by the macula densa and so actually eliminate the feedback signal (see Briggs and Schnermann in Suggested Readings).

[3] There are also some beta-adrenergic receptors on renal arteriolar smooth muscle, but so few in comparison to the alpha-adrenergic receptors that epinephrine causes only vasoconstriction in the kidneys.

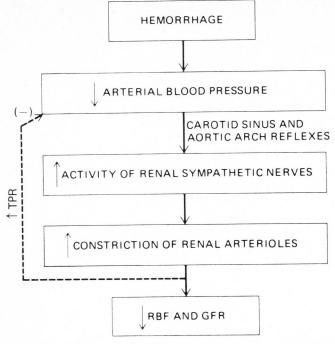

Figure 5-3 Pathway by which arterial hypotension causes, via arterial baroreceptors, reflex vasoconstriction mediated by the renal sympathetic nerves (epinephrine, released from the adrenal medulla, enhances the renal vasoconstriction). Decreases in venous and cardiac pressures also elicit, via baroreceptors in these structures, the same response. The increased renal resistance not only lowers RBF and GFR but also helps to restore blood pressure (the negative-feedback loop) by contributing to increased total peripheral resistance (TPR).

carotid sinus and aortic arch baroreceptors (Fig. 5-3). This sympathetic input causes renal afferent- and efferent-arteriolar constriction, which decreases RBF. Thus, although autoregulation blunts the *direct* effects on the kidney of changes in arterial pressure, **sympathetic reflexes** can still cause changes in renal hemodynamics when systemic arterial pressure is altered.

A second fact is that these reflexes also decrease GFR, although not to the same extent as RBF decreases. The major reason for the decrease in GFR during enhanced sympathetic outflow to the kidneys is the increase in afferent-arteriolar constriction induced by this input: Afferent-arteriolar constriction → increased afferent-arteriolar resistance → decreased glomerular-capillary hydraulic pressure → decreased GFR.

If sympathetic input were solely to the afferent arteriole, the decreases in GFR and RBF induced by increased sympathetic tone would be approximately proportional. However, both afferent and efferent arterioles receive sympathetic innervation and are constricted, though not to the same degree, when sympathetic tone is increased. Therefore, GFR tends not to decrease as much as RBF decreases. As described in Chap. 2,

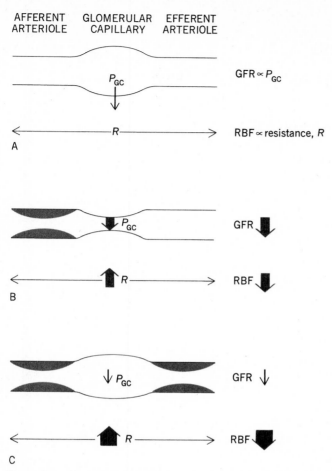

AFFERENT   GLOMERULAR   EFFERENT
ARTERIOLE   CAPILLARY   ARTERIOLE

P_{GC} $GFR \propto P_{GC}$

$\longleftarrow\qquad R\qquad\longrightarrow$ $RBF \propto$ resistance, R

A

P_{GC} GFR

R RBF

B

$\downarrow P_{GC}$ GFR $\downarrow$

R RBF

C

Figure 5-4 Effects of afferent-arteriolar constriction (B) and combined afferent-efferent-arteriolar constriction (C) on GFR and RBF. Adding efferent constriction to afferent constriction lowers RBF still further (because total resistance is increased) but restores GFR toward normal. The filtration fraction, GFR/RBF, is therefore increased.

the reason for this result is that because the efferent arterioles lie beyond the glomerulus, an increase in their resistance tends to *raise* glomerular-capillary pressure—just the opposite of the effect of afferent-arteriolar constriction (Fig. 5-4). In other words, sympathetically induced afferent and efferent constriction induce opposing effects on glomerular-capillary pressure—and, hence, GFR—but additive effects on renal vascular resistance—and, hence, RBF.

Because GFR decreases relatively less than RBF, the filtration fraction—GFR/RPF—increases. We shall make use of this fact in Chap. 7, when the control of salt and water excretion is described.

What is the adaptive value of this sympathetically mediated renal vasoconstriction triggered by a decrease in systemic arterial blood pressure? For one thing, it is simply a component of the rapidly occurring general homeostatic regulation of arterial pressure. The renal vasoconstriction contributes to a rise in total peripheral resistance, which helps rapidly restore the arterial blood pressure toward normal (Fig. 5-3). But there is a second, less obvious, way in which renal vasoconstriction helps raise arterial pressure, namely, lowering the excretion of sodium and water. Renal vasoconstriction achieves a reduction in salt and water excretion both by lowering GFR (and, hence, the filtered load of these substances) and, as we shall see in Chap. 7, by increasing tubular reabsorption of these substances.

Finally, it should be emphasized that although this entire discussion has been in terms of the renal response to *arterial* hypotension, the same type of sympathetically mediated vasoconstriction can also be triggered by baroreceptors in the veins or cardiac chambers. Indeed input from these baroreceptors probably has greater reflex effects on the renal circulation than does input from the arterial baroreceptors. Input from the peripheral chemoreceptors (responding to hypoxia) or from higher brain centers (e.g., during heavy exercise or emotional situations) also can trigger increased sympathetic outflow to the kidneys.

ANGIOTENSIN II

A second major regulator of the renal circulation is the renin-angiotensin system. Angiotensin II is a powerful vasoconstrictor, and the renal arterioles are quite sensitive to it. This hormone, like norephinephrine and epinephrine, constricts both afferent and efferent arterioles[4] and therefore also produces a lesser decrease in GFR than in RBF, resulting in an increase in filtration fraction.

Indeed, the efferent effect is so predominant that were the actions of angiotensin II on renal arterioles the only factor to be considered, little change in GFR would occur. In addition to these actions on renal arterioles, however, angiotensin II causes contraction of glomerular mesangial cells, which results in a decrease in K_f, an additional factor contributing to a decrease in GFR.

As described in Chap. 1, the plasma concentration of angiotensin II is increased when the kidneys are stimulated to secrete more renin; accordingly, angiotensin-induced renal hemodynamic changes can be expected whenever renin secretion is significantly elevated.

---

[4] Although there is considerable controversy over whether angiotensin II exerts any effect at all on afferent arterioles, I believe the evidence favors the conclusion that this hormone normally does act on both sets of arterioles, although to a greater extent on the efferent arteriole (see Navar in Suggested Readings).

Control of Renin Secretion

At this point, the student should review the basic biochemistry of the renin-angiotensin system and the anatomy of the juxtaglomerular apparatus, both described in Chap. 1. The control of renin secretion is quite complex since there are at least four major types of inputs, which are strongly interrelated with one another.[5] These four mechanisms are (1) an intrarenal baroreceptor, (2) a tubular sodium or chloride receptor in the macula densa, (3) the renal sympathetic nerves, and (4) angiotensin II itself.

Intrarenal Baroreceptors   The renin-secreting granular cells themselves act as **intrarenal baroreceptors**, i.e., as pressure or distention receptors, monitoring the pressure or vascular volume within the last portions of the afferent arterioles (Fig.1-3) and varying their secretion of renin *inversely* with these parameters. This makes good sense teleologically. For example, consider the response to hemorrhage (Fig. 5-5): The pressure at the juxtaglomerular ends of the afferent arterioles is reduced both because of decreased arterial pressure and because of reflexly increased sympathetic outflow to the arterioles. This decreased arteriolar pressure causes less stretch of the JG cells and, hence, increased release of renin from the granular cells.

Macula Densa   Earlier in this chapter, we described how the macula densa is involved in autoregulation of GFR via tubuloglomerular feedback. Now we describe here another completely distinct function for the macula densa—control of renin secretion.

In discussing tubuloglomerular feedback, we pointed out that an increased flow to the macula densa is accompanied by increased sodium and chloride concentrations in the macula densa lumen and, hence, increased sodium chloride reabsorption by the cells. We stated that this increased reabsorption somehow generates the signal for *increased* production of a vasoconstrictor. Now we point out that this same signal elicits *inhibition* of renin release.[6] Such a reflex makes sense teleologically since it is simply a logical extension of the reflex described for the intrarenal baroreceptor (Fig. 5-6).

---

[5] Despite the complexity, there is probably a final common pathway for all inputs controlling renin release—cytosolic calcium concentration. Increased cytosolic calcium concentration in the granular cells (or possibly one of the other JGA cell types) inhibits renin release, whereas decreased calcium concentration stimulates it. (See Churchill in Suggested Readings.)

[6] Note that renin release and, hence, angiotensin II formation is low when the production of the vasoconstrictor mediating tubuloglomerular feedback is high. This is strong evidence that angiotensin II does not mediate tubuloglomerular feedback.

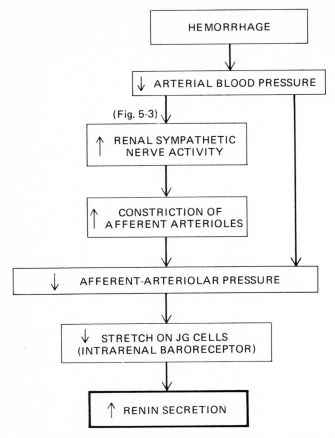

Figure 5-5 Intrarenal baroreceptor control of renin secretion during hemorrhage.

Renal Sympathetic Nerves   We have already described one important mechanism by which increased renal sympathetic nerve activity (and increased circulating epinephrine) results in an increase of renin secretion, namely, by causing constriction of the afferent arterioles. This stimulates the intrarenal baroreceptor by reducing the hydraulic pressure at the end of the afferent arteriole (Fig. 5-5), and it also stimulates the macula densa receptor by reducing flow to the macula densa (Fig. 5-6). In this manner, the renal sympathetic nerves play *indirect* roles in controlling renin secretion.

In addition, however, sympathetic neurons end in the immediate vicinity of the granular cells (Fig. 5-7), and these neurons exert a *direct* stimulatory effect on renin secretion via beta$_1$-adrenergic receptors on the granular cells. Actually, this direct effect is more sensitive than the indirect ones involving the intrarenal baroreceptor and macula densa

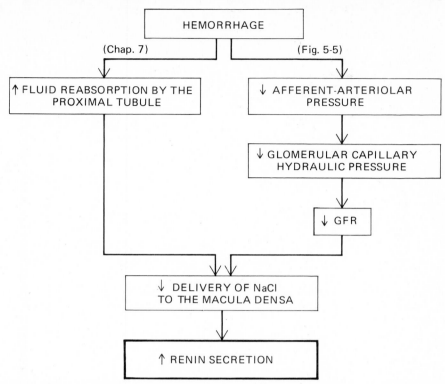

Figure 5-6 Macula densa control of renin secretion during hemorrhage. The pathway leading to decreased GFR is merely a continuation of Fig. 5-5. The mechanisms by which hemorrhage enhances fluid reabsorption by the proximal tubule are described in Chap. 7.

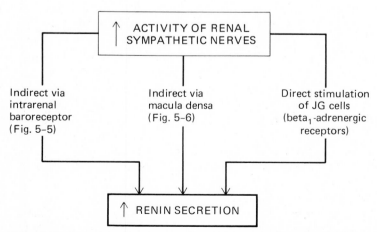

Figure 5-7 Summary of mechanisms by which increased renal sympathetic outflow causes increased renin secretion. The direct effect is probably the most important of these pathways.

since increases in sympathetic outflow to the kidneys too small to elicit vasoconstriction or altered flow to the macula densa still cause increased renin secretion.

Angiotensin II   Angiotensin II exerts a direct inhibitory effect on renin secretion by the granular cells. This is an example of a negative feedback in which a hormone inhibits the secretion of its own stimulating substance, analogous to the inhibition of ACTH secretion by cortisol or to inhibition of TSH secretion by thyroxine. By this mechanism, angiotensin II exerts a dampening effect on its own rate of production.

Other Inputs Controlling Renin Release   There are many inputs other than the four just described that have been shown to be capable of altering renin release. These include, among others, ADH, potassium, and calcium, all of which can inhibit renin release. The physiological significance of these pathways is mainly that they provide additional loops in the feedback mechanisms integrating the metabolism of sodium with that of water and the other ions. Under most circumstances, they are of only minor importance, but this may not be true in clinical situations characterized by a large excess or deficit of any of them.[7]

PROSTAGLANDINS

Several of the renally produced prostaglandins (the more general term for these substances is *eicosanoids*), notably **PGE_2** and **PGI_2,** are vasodilators, particularly of the afferent arterioles. The best documented physiological role for these vasodilator prostaglandins is to dampen the vasoconstrictor effect of the renal nerves and angiotensin II. Increased activity of the renal nerves or increased plasma angiotensin II stimulates the kidney to synthesize and release vasodilator prostaglandins. The end result is that much of the vasoconstrictor actions of norepinephrine and angiotensin II are counteracted by the vasodilator action of the prostaglandins, and the renal resistance changes much less than would otherwise have occurred (Fig. 5-8).[8] Vasodilator prostaglandins oppose not

---

[7] Of particular interest is yet another input—renal prostaglandins. Several of the prostaglandins produced within the kidneys, notably PGE_2 and PGI_2, can stimulate renin secretion, and these prostaglandins act as mediators or modulators of certain of the other inputs. Present evidence suggests that beta-adrenergic control over renin secretion is independent of prostaglandins but that the prostaglandins are somehow involved in, although probably not absolutely essential for, the macula densa and intrarenal-baroreceptor pathways (see Keeton and Campbell in Suggested Readings).

[8] If one puts the information in this section and in footnote 7 together, it is apparent that a potential positive feedback mechanism exists between prostaglandins and the renin-angiotensin system: ↑ renin release → ↑ [renin] → ↑ [angiotensin II] → ↑ PG release → ↑ [PG] → ↑ renin release → etc. Whether such a positive feedback mechanism does, in fact, ever occur will remain unclear until we know more about the exact identities and sites of production of the various prostaglandins that interact with the renin-angiotensin system.

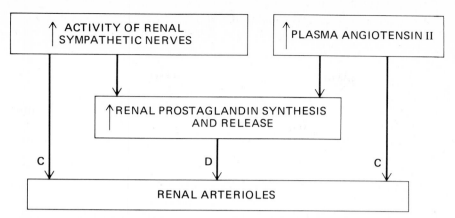

Figure 5-8 "Dampening" effect of prostaglandins on renal vasoconstriction induced by the renal nerves or angiotensin II (C = constriction; D = dilation).

only the arteriolar effects of angiotensin II but the mesangial-constricting effects as well.

If we return once more to our example of hypotension because of hemorrhage, we see that three factors are reducing renal blood flow and GFR—the decreased blood pressure per se, the renal sympathetic nerves, and angiotensin II. Simultaneously, two factors are minimizing the reduction—autoregulation and the vasodilator prostaglandins, whose release is stimulated by the renal nerves and angiotensin II. The net result is usually a modest increase in renal vascular resistance, leading to a modest decrease in RBF and GFR. The adaptive value of having such opposing inputs is to strike a balance between, on the one hand, the requirement for an increased total peripheral resistance to maintain systemic arterial pressure (for the "benefit" of the heart and brain) and, on the other hand, the likelihood of renal damage if renal vasoconstriction were too severe. For example, an experimental animal given a drug that blocks prostaglandin synthesis and then subjected to even a modest hemorrhage may suffer rapid, severe renal damage because of a profound reduction in renal blood flow.

The kidneys also produce several vasoconstrictor prostaglandins, notably TXA_2. No physiological role has yet been demonstrated for these vasoconstrictors. However, certain disease states (e.g., ureteral obstruction and drug-induced acute renal failure) are associated with an increased intrarenal production of TXA_2, which may be a major cause of the intense and harmful vasoconstriction seen in these states.

OTHER FACTORS

The renal vasculature is sensitive to many other naturally occurring chemical messengers. The posterior pituitary hormone, **antidiuretic hor-**

mone (vasopressin), when present in high plasma concentrations, causes both renal vasoconstriction and mesangial-cell contraction, thereby lowering RBF and GFR. Antidiuretic hormone also stimulates release of prostaglandins that oppose its actions.

Dopamine, in contrast to vasopressin, is a renal vasodilator, and there is some evidence, as noted in Chap. 1, for the existence of renal-sympathetic-dopaminergic neurons. The intrarenally produced kinins (Chap. 1) are also potent vasodilators, and adenosine (mentioned earlier as a possible mediator for tubuloglomerular feedback) is a renal vaso-constrictor. However, whether dopamine, the kinins, and adenosine actually play significant roles in the control of renal hemodynamics remains to be determined.

INTRARENAL DISTRIBUTION OF BLOOD FLOW

The cortex receives more than 90 percent of the total renal blood flow. The paucity of medullary blood flow (its adaptive value for urine concentration will be discussed later) is due to the high resistance offered by the vasa recta.

There are also differences in the relative distribution of blood flow within the cortex among the juxtamedullary, midcortical, and superficial cortical nephrons. The physiological significance of this heterogeneity is still unknown.

Study questions: 28 to 33

6

BASIC RENAL PROCESSES FOR SODIUM, CHLORIDE, AND WATER

OBJECTIVES

The student constructs typical balance sheets for total-body water and total-body sodium chloride

The student understands the basic renal processes for sodium, chloride, and water.

1 Summarizes the three generalizations that apply to sodium, chloride, and water reabsorption along the tubule
2 Describes the basic pathways for sodium and water reabsorption, including fluid movement into peritubular capillaries, and the coupling between them
3 States the driving forces for passive and active chloride reabsorption
4 Calculates or lists the quantities of sodium, chloride, and water normally filtered, reabsorbed, and excreted per day

The student understands the mechanisms of sodium, chloride, and water reabsorption in each tubular segment.

1 Describes the major transport process for each of these substances in each tubular segment and the interrelationships between them; defines transtubular PD and gives its orientation in the different tubular segments
2 States the differences in ion transport between the early and the mid-to-late portions of the proximal tubule
3 Describes the changes in the concentrations of the major ions and organic solutes along the length of the proximal tubule
4 Describes the mechanism of action of osmotic diuretics
5 States the fluid osmolarity and relative water permeability in each nephron segment during water diuresis and antidiuresis
6 Lists the percentages of sodium and water reabsorbed by each nephron segment during antidiuresis and water diuresis
7 Describes the countercurrent multiplier system for urine concentration; states the transport and permeability characteristics of the ascending and descending limbs, the distal convoluted tubules, and the collecting-duct system
8 States the net loss or gain of solute and water for the two limbs of the loop and the collecting duct; states the action of ADH and the nephron sites on which it acts; describes the interaction of ADH and prostaglandins

9 Describes how urea diffusion out of the inner medullary collecting ducts contributes to urine concentrating ability
10 Describes the medullary circulation and its functioning as a countercurrent exchanger
11 States how changes in medullary blood-flow or loop-flow rates may impede concentration of the urine
12 Describes the obligatory relationships between sodium and water excretion; states how the tubular segments differ in their ability to develop transtubular sodium gradients

   A balance sheet for total-body water is given in Table 6-1. It should be recognized that these are average values, which are subject to considerable variation. The two sources of body water are metabolically produced water, resulting largely from the oxidation of carbohydrates, and ingested water, obtained from liquids and so-called solid food (a rare steak is approximately 70 percent water). There are four sites from which water is always lost to the external environment: skin, lungs, gastrointestinal tract, and kidneys. Menstrual flow constitutes a fifth potential source of water loss in women. The loss of water by evaporation from the cells of the skin and the lining of respiratory passageways is a continuous process, often referred to as **insensible loss** because the person is unaware of its occurrence. Additional water can be made available for evaporation from the skin by the production of sweat. Fecal water loss is normally quite small but can be severe in diarrhea. Gastrointestinal loss can also be large in vomiting.

   Table 6-2 is a typical balance sheet for sodium and chloride. The excretion of sodium and chloride via the skin and gastrointestinal tract is normally quite small but may increase markedly during severe sweating, burns, vomiting, or diarrhea. Hemorrhage can also result in the loss of large quantities of both salt and water.

Table 6-1   Normal Routes of Water Gain and Loss in Adults

Route	mL/day
Intake	
Drunk	1200
In food	1000
Metabolically produced	350
Total	2550
Output	
Insensible loss (skin and lungs)	900
Sweat	50
In feces	100
Urine	1500
Total	2550

Table 6-2   Normal Routes of
Sodium Chloride Intake and Loss

Route	g/day
Intake	
Food	10.5
Output	
Sweat	0.25
Feces	0.25
Urine	10.0
Total output	10.5

Control of the renal excretion of sodium, chloride, and water constitutes the most important mechanism for the regulation of the body content of these substances. Their excretory rates can be varied over an extremely wide range. For example, a consumer of gross amounts of salt may ingest 20 to 25 g of sodium chloride per day, whereas a person on a low-salt diet may ingest only 50 mg. The normal kidney can readily alter its excretion of salt over this range. Similarly, urinary water excretion can be varied physiologically from approximately 400 mL/day to 25 L/day, depending on whether one is lost in the desert or participating in a beer-drinking contest.

Being of low molecular weight and not bound to protein, sodium, chloride, and water are all freely filterable at the renal corpuscle. They all undergo considerable tubular reabsorption—normally, more than 99 percent (see Table 2-3)—but no tubular secretion. Most renal energy is utilized to accomplish this enormous reabsorptive task.

The major tubular mechanisms for reabsorption of these substances can be summarized by three generalizations: (1) The reabsorption of sodium is mainly a primary active process dependent on the Na,K-ATPase pumps in the basolateral membrane. (2) The reabsorption of chloride may be passive or active, depending on the nephron segment, but in either case most chloride reabsorption is coupled in one way or another with primary active reabsorption of sodium. (3) The reabsorption of water is passive—osmosis—and depends on solute reabsorption, particularly sodium reabsorption. Thus, primary active tubular sodium reabsorption is the event that results in reabsorption of most chloride as well as water.

SODIUM REABSORPTION AND SODIUM-WATER COUPLING

We described in Chap. 2 how most sodium reabsorption is active and transcellular. Let us go over this pathway again, this time adding the passive reabsorption of water coupled to sodium reabsorption.

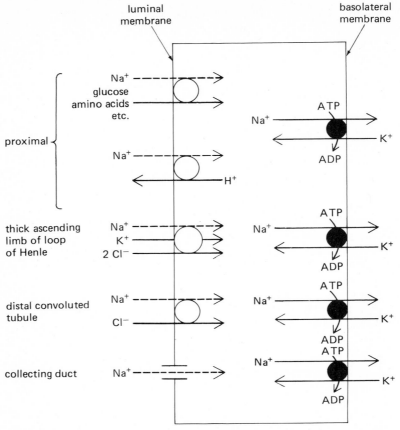

Figure 6-1 Mechanisms of sodium reabsorption along the tubule. Depending on the tubular segment, the step from lumen to cell is either by diffusion through channels or by carrier-mediated facilitated diffusion in which other substances are cotransported or countertransported with the sodium. In all cases the sodium movement across the luminal membrane is always "downhill." The "uphill" step across the basolateral membrane is via Na-K-ATPase "pumping" in all tubular segments. At the left, only the most common types of entry are shown for different tubular segments, and this categorization is not meant to be complete.

Recall that luminal sodium ions enter the cell along their electrochemical gradient (Fig. 2-7); the inside of the cell is negatively charged with respect to the lumen, and the intracellular sodium concentration is low because of the active transport of sodium, by the Na,K-ATPase, across the basolateral membrane into the interstitial fluid. Depending on the tubular segment (Fig. 6-1), sodium's "downhill" movement from lumen into cell may be solely as sodium ions through sodium channels, as cotransport with other substances (glucose, amino acids, chloride, etc.), or as countertransport with hydrogen ion, but the "uphill" step from cell to interstitial fluid is always via the Na,K-ATPase pumps.

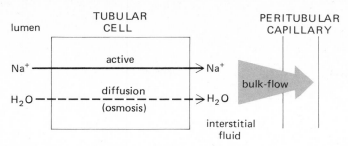

Figure 6-2 Coupling of water and sodium reabsorption. Reabsorption of sodium creates a difference in osmolarity between lumen and interstitial fluid, which causes the diffusion (osmosis) of water in the same direction. The water moves both through and between cells (the latter via the tight junctions). Movement of both solute and water from interstitial fluid into peritubular capillaries occurs by bulk flow.

Now for water reabsorption: The movement of sodium from lumen to interstitial fluid *lowers* total luminal osmolarity (i.e., raises water concentration) and simultaneously *raises* the osmolarity (lowers the water concentration) in the interstitial fluid. This osmotic gradient from lumen to intercellular space causes net diffusion of water from the lumen across the plasma membranes and/or tight junctions into the interstitial fluid (Fig. 6–2). Just how much net osmosis will occur under any given lumen-to-interstitium osmotic gradient is determined by the permeability to water of the plasma membranes and tight junctions. As we shall see, this permeability varies along the nephron and is subject to physiological control.

To generalize, water reabsorption is due to the differences in osmolarity between lumen and interstitial fluid created by reabsorption of solute.[1] We have mentioned only sodium reabsorption, but the reabsorption of other solutes also contributes to differences in osmolarity and, hence, water reabsorption. However, the reabsorption of most of these other solutes is, itself, ultimately ascribable to sodium reabsorption (Table 6-3). In Chap. 4 we saw that this is true for the many organic substances actively reabsorbed proximally by cotransport with sodium. We shall see, in subsequent sections, that it is also true for most chloride reabsorption and most bicarbonate reabsorption; these are, quantitatively, the only important inorganic anions.

We have been describing only the movements of sodium and water out of the lumen and into the interstitial fluid. What causes this reabsorbed fluid to move from interstitial fluid into peritubular capillaries

[1] To be more accurate, one should refer not to differences in *absolute* osmolarity but to differences in *effective* osmolarity. Because of differences in the reflection coefficients of different solutes, it is quite possible to have transtubular differences in effective osmolarity in the absence of differences in absolute osmolarity. For a discussion of this complexity with regard to proximal water reabsorption, see articles by Schafer in Suggested Readings.

Table 6-3   Summary of Mechanisms by Which Reabsorption of Sodium Drives Reabsorption of Other Substances

Reabsorption of sodium:
1. Creates lumen-negative transtubular potential difference across the epithelium, and this favors paracellular reabsorption of anions (e.g., chloride) by diffusion
2. Creates transtubular osmolarity difference, which favors reabsorption of water by osmosis; in turn water reabsorpton concentrates many luminal solutes (e.g., chloride and urea), thereby favoring their reabsorption by diffusion
3. Achieves reabsorption of many organic nutrients, phosphate, and chloride by cotransport
4. Achieves secretion of hydrogen ion (in the proximal tubule) by countertransport; these hydrogen ions are required for reabsorption of bicarbonate (as described in Chap. 9)

(Fig. 6-2)? It is, simply, bulk-flow caused by the net balance of hydraulic and oncotic pressures acting across the peritubular capillaries.

Net pressure for fluid movement from interstitium into peritubular capillaries is given by the following equation:

$$P_{net} = P_{Int} + \pi_{PC} - P_{PC} - \pi_{Int}$$

where P = hydraulic pressure, π = oncotic pressure, and the subscripts Int and PC stand for interstitium and peritubular capillary. This is the second time we have dealt with capillary dynamics in the kidney, the first being the discussion of glomerular filtration. It must be emphasized that the concepts are identical, but of course the locations are different. Glomerular dynamics involves the balance of forces between the glomerular capillaries and Bowman's capsule, whereas the peritubular forces are between the interstitium and the peritubular capillaries. Representative numbers are given for these forces in Table 6-4; the exact numbers are not important or worth memorizing (indeed, precise values are not available for the human kidney) but are given only to illustrate the following basic principles.

Whereas the net driving pressure across the glomerular membranes always favors filtration *out of* the capillaries into Bowman's capsule, the net driving pressure across the peritubular capillaries always favors net movement *into* the capillaries. The major reason for the latter fact is twofold: (1) The peritubular-capillary hydraulic pressure is generally quite low (10 to 15 mmHg) because the blood entering the peritubular capillaries has already had to flow through the afferent arterioles, glomeruli, and efferent arterioles. (2) The oncotic pressure of the plasma entering the peritubular capillaries is higher than that of the plasma entering the glomerular capillaries because the plasma proteins are concentrated by loss of protein-free filtrate during passage through the glomerular capillaries. Early peritubular-capillary oncotic pressure is, therefore, identical to end glomerular-capillary oncotic pressure.

Table 6-4   Estimated Forces Involved in Movement of Fluid from Interstitium into Peritubular Capillaries*

Forces	mmHg
1 Favoring uptake	
a Interstitial hydraulic pressure, P_{Int}	3
b Oncotic pressure in peritubular capillaries, π_{PC}	33
2 Opposing uptake	
a Hydraulic pressure in peritubular capillaries, P_{PC}	15
b Interstitial oncotic pressure, π_{Int}	6
3 Net pressure for uptake (1 − 2)	15

* The values for peritubular-capillary hydraulic and oncotic pressures are for the early portions of the capillary. The oncotic pressure, of course, decreases as protein-free fluid enters it, i.e., as absorption occurs, but would not go below 25 mmHg (the value of arterial plasma) even if all fluid originally filtered at the glomerulus were absorbed.

CHLORIDE REABSORPTION

As stated earlier, chloride reabsorption can be either passive or active. How is the *passive* reabsorption of chloride coupled to the active transport of sodium? There are at least two mechanisms responsible for this coupling (Fig. 6-3). The first mechanism is precisely the same as that previously described for urea. As water moves out of the tubule secondary to sodium reabsorption, all solutes in the tubule not subject to active reabsorption will increase in concentration. By this means, a chloride *concentration gradient* is established across the tubular epithelium and acts as a driving force for paracellular chloride reabsorption. (You should now recognize that the reabsorption of urea, just as that of chloride, ultimately depends on sodium reabsorption via the latter's effect on water reabsorption.)

The second mechanism coupling *passive* chloride reabsorption to active sodium reabsorption is the **electric potential difference (PD)** that exists across the tubular epithelium. In several tubular segments (we shall be more specific later), the tubular lumen is negatively charged compared to the interstitial fluid. The major factor contributing to this potential is the active reabsorption of sodium. Just on an intuitive level, it should be evident that the active transport of positively charged sodium ions across the epithelium tends to leave the inside of the lumen negatively charged with respect to the interstitial fluid. A systematic analysis of the precise origins of this transtubular PD is beyond the scope of this presentation. What is important for present purposes is the fact that this PD exists in several tubular segments, is contributed to by active sodium transport, and constitutes a driving force for paracellular chloride reabsorption by diffusion.

Depending on the tubular segment, therefore, there is an electric and/or a chemical (i.e., concentration) difference favoring passive chloride reabsorption. In the proximal tubule, where the PD is very small and may actually be slightly lumen-positive in its late portions, the concentration difference created by sodium-coupled water transport is the impor-

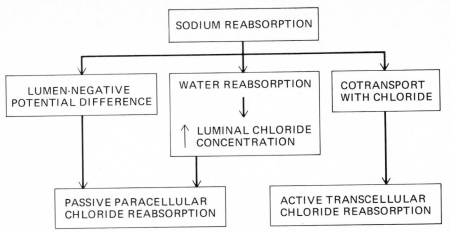

Figure 6-3 *Mechanisms by which chloride reabsorption, whether passive or active, is coupled to sodium reabsorption. See Table 6-5 for application of these mechanisms to specific tubular segments.*

tant factor. In the distal convoluted tubules and portions of the collecting ducts, a very large lumen-negative PD exists and constitutes the major driving force for passive chloride movement.

Thus far we have described only the *passive* reabsorption of chloride. In several tubular segments (again, we shall be more specific later), there also exist *secondary active reabsorptive processes* for chloride. The most important, quantitatively, of these involves cotransport of the chloride with sodium across the luminal membrane.

With these generalizations as guides, let us now discuss some of the distinct characteristics of the individual tubular segments relative to salt and water handling. But first a word or two of explanation (or apology) is in order. First, for simplicity, these sections on the individual tubular segments give only those transport mechanisms that are quantitatively most important; additional processes exist, some of which are mentioned in the footnotes, and the interested reader can consult the Suggested Readings for more information. Second, since chloride transport is, with one exception, always dependent ultimately on sodium transport, one might question the value of presenting the individual chloride mechanisms; however, an understanding of the various drugs that are used clinically as diuretics often depends on distinguishing these different pathways.

PROXIMAL TUBULE

The proximal tubule (including both the convoluted and straight portions) is the site of greatest sodium, chloride, and water reabsorption. Approximately 65 percent of the filtered sodium and water and a somewhat

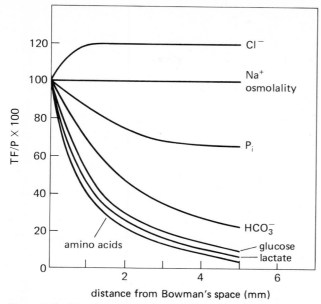

Figure 6-4 Changes in tubular fluid composition along the proximal convoluted tubule. TF = the concentration of the substance in tubular fluid; P = its concentration in arterial plasma. Values below unity indicate that relatively more of the substance than of water has been reabsorbed; values above unity indicate that relatively less of the substance than water has been reabsorbed. (*Figure modified from FC Rector, Am J Physiol 1983; 249: F461; and from DA Maddox and JF Gennari, Am J Physiol 1987; 252: F573.*)

smaller fraction of filtered chloride are reabsorbed by the time the fluid has reached the end of the proximal tubule.

The proximal reabsorption of sodium is, of course, mainly a primary active process, driven by the Na,K-ATPase pumps in the basolateral membrane.[2] Let us look more closely at the luminal entry steps (Fig. 6-1). In the early portion, a large fraction of the sodium entering the cell across the luminal membrane enters via cotransport with organic nutrients and phosphate, the luminal concentrations of which decrease rapidly (Fig. 6-4). The rest of the sodium movement from the lumen into the cell in the early proximal tubule is mainly via countertransport with hydrogen ion; i.e., as sodium ions enter the cell, hydrogen ions are secreted uphill by the same carrier into the lumen. As will be described in Chap. 9, these hydrogen ions drive the secondary active reabsorption of filtered bicar-

---

[2] The reason for the word *mainly* in this statement and several times previously is that in late portions of the proximal tubule, some paracellular sodium reabsorption occurs by passive processes—both simple diffusion and solvent drag. I have chosen not to describe this phenomenon in the text because these passive pathways constitute a minor fraction of total proximal sodium reabsorption and because the forces driving them owe their existence ultimately to the usual active sodium transport occurring in earlier proximal segments. (See articles by Schafer in Suggested Readings.) (See footnote 4 for a continuation of this subject.)

bonate. Thus, in the early proximal tubule, bicarbonate is the major anion reabsorbed with sodium, and luminal bicarbonate falls significantly (Fig. 6-4).

What about chloride reabsorption? It is mainly passive along the entire proximal tubule.[3] Along the early proximal tubule, the reabsorption of water, driven by reabsorption of sodium plus its cotransported solutes and bicarbonate, causes luminal chloride concentrations to increase substantially (Fig. 6-4). Accordingly, as the fluid flows through the middle and late proximal tubule, this concentration gradient, maintained by continued water reabsorption, provides the major driving force for passive paracellular chloride reabsorption. Thus, in the middle and late proximal tubule, chloride becomes the major substance reabsorbed with sodium.[4]

What is the sodium concentration and osmolarity along the proximal tubule? As shown in Fig. 6-4, both these parameters remain essentially equal to their values in plasma. This fact may come as a surprise to you since you might logically (but wrongly, in this case) assume that sodium concentration would decrease markedly as its reabsorption proceeds. But remember that we are dealing here with sodium *concentration*. The water permeability of the proximal tubule is so great that passive water reabsorption keeps pace with active sodium reabsorption. Thus, whereas 65 percent of the *mass* of filtered sodium has been reabsorbed by the end of the proximal tubule, so has almost the same percentage of filtered water. Therefore, the concentration of sodium, as opposed to the mass, remains virtually unchanged during fluid passage through the proximal tubule.

To be more precise in the previous paragraph, we should have stated that water reabsorption keeps pace with *total solute* reabsorption, not just sodium reabsorption. But sodium and solutes whose reabsorption is coupled in one way or another to sodium reabsorption constitute the overwhelming majority of all solutes reabsorbed, and so we can use *sodium reabsorption* and *total solute reabsorption* almost interchangably in the proximal tubule.

Figure 6-4 summarizes the concentration changes along the proximal tubule that we have been describing; all these changes reflect the ratio of

---

[3] In addition, a significant fraction of chloride reabsorption in the proximal tubule is secondary active, involving anion countertransporters in the luminal membrane and possibly the peritubular membrane as well. This process is ultimately dependent on sodium reabsorption. (See Karniski and Aronson in Suggested Readings.)

[4] This passive reabsorptive movement of chloride down its electrochemical gradient may be so great in the late proximal tubule that it causes the lumen to become positively charged relative to the intersitium. This lumen-positive potential, in turn, provides a force driving passive reabsorption of sodium. Thus, as noted in footnote 2, a fraction of late proximal sodium reabsorption may normally be passive. But note that if you go back far enough, you will see that this passive reabsorption is traceable to active sodium reabsorption upstream, in the earlier proximal tubule (early proximal sodium reabsorption → early proximal water reabsorption → concentration of luminal chloride → diffusion of chloride out of later proximal tubule → lumen-positive PD → passive sodium reabsorption). (See articles by Schafer, and Schild and Giebisch, in Suggested Readings.)

that solute's reabsorption to water reabsorption. Sodium remains virtually identical to plasma. Bicarbonate becomes lower than in plasma, and chloride higher. Some organic solutes, like glucose, are lower, whereas some, like urea, are higher. The end result is that the total osmolarity—the sum of all individual solute concentrations—all along the proximal tubule is always essentially the same as that of plasma. This result, of course, is not just fortuitous but must be the case, given the extremely high permeability of the proximal tubule to water. In other words, water reabsorption always occurs at a rate that keeps the luminal osmolarity only very slighty less than that of the interstitial fluid and plasma. Indeed, the difference is so small as to be undetectable in most experiments.

Given the extremely high water permeability of proximal tubule to water, is there any way to break the tight coupling between sodium reabsorption and water reabsorption in this tubular segment? Let us administer to a dog large amounts of the carbohydrate mannitol so that its plasma concentration equals 100 mosmol/L. Mannitol is freely filtered at the renal corpuscle but is not reabsorbed. In the very first portion of the proximal tubule, therefore, mannitol will contribute 100 mosmol/L. As sodium is actively reabsorbed, the total osmolarity of the proximal-tubular fluid begins to decrease ever so slightly, and water, therefore, passively follows the sodium. However, because the mannitol cannot be reabsorbed, its concentration increases as water is reabsorbed. This type of concentrating effect has been previously described for chloride and for urea and obviously will apply to any solute whose reabsorption is slower than that of water.

The crucial difference between our experimental conditions and the normal state is that the normally present "lagging" solutes either are present in low concentrations or, like urea and chloride, follow the water to a relatively large degree. The mannitol, in contrast, is present in a very large concentration in our experiment and is not reabsorbed at all. Accordingly, as its concentration rises as a result of water reabsorption, its osmotic presence retards the further reabsorption of water. Thus, passive water movement is prevented from keeping up with active sodium transport. The result is that sodium concentration in the lumen decreases well below plasma sodium concentration.

Agents such as mannitol, in our example, that retard water reabsorption because of their osmotic contribution are called **osmotic diuretics.** Such agents, perhaps surprisingly to you at this moment, also cause the excretion of large quantities of sodium (and chloride), although to a lesser extent than of water. The major reason for this phenomenon illustrates another important characteristic of renal sodium transport: Simultaneously with the *active* transport of sodium out of the tubule, there are quite large paracellular fluxes of sodium in both directions by diffusion because the intercellular junctional complexes are quite permeable to sodium (recall that the proximal tubule is a "leaky" epithelium). But is there normally a *net diffusional flux* into or out of the proximal tubule? Normally there is almost none since there is no significant transtubular concentration difference for sodium and since the electric potential difference across the proximal tubule is quite small. Therefore, the opposing diffusional fluxes of sodium simply cancel each other out, leaving only the outwardly directed *active* sodium-transport pathway to account for overall *net* sodium movement. However, in the presence of an osmotic diuretic, this situation is altered; because the osmotic diuretic retards water reabsorption, active sodium reabsorption causes the luminal sodium concentration to decrease as described above. As a result there is a sodium concentration gradient favoring *net diffusion* of sodium from interstitial fluid to lumen. This net passive paracellular influx opposes the active transcellular outflux, and so the *overall net* removal of sodium from the proximal-tubular lumen is diminished. This is one of the reasons that osmotic diuretics such as mannitol induce the excretion of large quantities of sodium (and chloride) as well as water.

The impression should not be left that osmotic diuretics inhibit water and electrolyte reabsorption in the proximal tubule only. In fact, major inhibition also occurs in the loop of Henle (although the mechanism is not exactly the same).

Osmotic diuresis occurs in several diseases, including severe diabetes mellitus. Glucose, as we have seen, is normally completely reabsorbed in the proximal tubule. But in patients with uncontrolled diabetes mellitus, the filtered load may exceed the glucose T_m, and large quantities of glucose may remain unreabsorbed. Just like mannitol in the preceding example, the glucose retards water and sodium reabsorption and causes an osmotic diuresis. In such a patient, the filtered load of the ketone bodies, acetoacetate and β-hydroxybutyrate, may also exceed the T_ms for these substances so that they also contribute to the osmotic diuresis.

LOOP OF HENLE

The loop of Henle normally reabsorbs approximately 25 percent of the filtered sodium and chloride and 15 percent of the filtered water. Thus, unlike the proximal tubule, the loop of Henle reabsorbs proportionally more sodium chloride than water.

There is also an extremely important geographic separation of sodium chloride reabsorption and water reabsorption. The descending loop of Henle (DLH) does not reabsorb sodium or chloride but does reabsorb water. In contrast, the ascending loop of Henle (ALH) reabsorbs sodium and chloride but little, if any, water. The DLH seems to violate our generalization that water reabsorption occurs as a passive consequence of

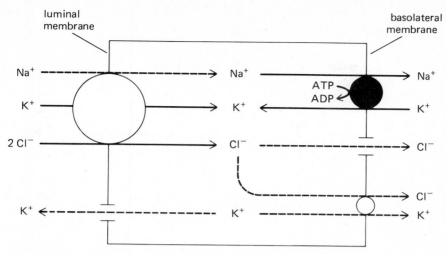

Figure 6-5 Model of transcellular electrolyte transport by the thick ascending loop of Henle. Broken lines indicate downhill transport, and solid lines indicate active transport, either primary or secondary. Note that potassium is basically recycled at both the luminal and basolateral membranes, whereas the cell achieves net reabsorption of both sodium and chloride.

sodium reabsorption, but it does not. However, because water reabsorption in this segment is so tied up with events occuring beyond the loop, we will delay resolving how the DLH can reabsorb water even though it does not reabsorb sodium until we have described these more distal segments. For now we will simply describe ALH sodium and chloride reabsorption.

The mechanisms of sodium and chloride reabsorption by the thin ALH, in contrast to the thick ALH, are still unclear, as will be discussed below. In the thick ALH, the reabsorption of sodium is mainly a primary active process dependent, as elsewhere, on Na,K-ATPase pumps in the basolateral membrane.[5] The luminal entry step for sodium in this segment is by cotransport with potassium and chloride, and the carrier is termed a Na,K,2Cl cotransporter. This cotransporter achieves the secondary active reabsorption of chloride and is the major pathway for chloride reabsorption in this segment. Figure 6-5 summarizes ion transport by the thick ALH.

[5] It has been estimated, however, that as much as 50 percent of sodium reabsorption in this segment may be by paracellular diffusion. There is a high paracellular conduction for sodium in the thick ALH, and the lumen-positive potential in this segment is a significant driving force for passive sodium reabsorption. Again, as in the case for the proximal tubule (footnote 4), any such passive sodium reabsorption depends ultimately on Na,K-ATPase activity to set up the lumen-positive potential. (See articles by Greger and by Molony et al. in Suggested Readings.)

DISTAL CONVOLUTED TUBULE
AND COLLECTING-DUCT SYSTEM

By the end of the ALH, only about 10 percent of the originally filtered sodium and chloride and 20 percent of the filtered water still remain in the tubule, the rest having been reabsorbed by the proximal tubule and loop of Henle.

Sodium and chloride reabsorption continues along the distal convoluted tubule and collecting-duct system so that the final urine normally contains less than 1 percent of the total filtered sodium and chloride. More important than this vague single value—less than 1 percent—is the fact that the exact number is homeostatically regulated, largely by the adrenocortical hormone, **aldosterone,** depending on the individual's salt balance, as we shall see in the next chapter.

The mechanism of sodium reabsorption is, as always, primary active transport. Its luminal entry step in the distal convoluted tubule is via Na,Cl cotransport (Fig. 6-1); this cotransporter has characteristics that differ significantly from the Na,K,2Cl cotransporter in the thick ALH and so is sensitive to different drugs. In the collecting-duct system, the luminal entry step for sodium is via sodium channels (Fig. 6-1).

Chloride reabsorption is both passive, driven by the large lumen-negative transtubular potential in these segments, and secondary active. The active component is achieved in the distal convoluted tubule by the luminal Na,Cl cotransporter noted above and in the cortical collecting duct by a luminal Cl,HCO_3 countertransporter. This countertransporter is the only significant mechanism for chloride reabsorption not coupled directly or indirectly with sodium reabsorption. The secondary active systems for chloride reabsorption in the distal convoluted tubule and cortical collecting duct are important for reabsorbing the last bit of chloride from the tubular fluid in states of bodily chloride deficiency.

This completes our summary of tubular chloride reabsorption, which is summarized in Table 6-5.

What about reabsorption of water in these tubular segments? The water permeability of the distal convoluted tubule is extremely low and unchanging. Accordingly, almost no water is reabsorbed during passage of fluid through it. In contrast, the water permeability of the collecting-duct system is subject to physiological control (see below) and may vary from extremely low to fairly high (although never as high as that of the proximal tubule).

Let us now combine the information on salt reabsorption and water permeability in following the changes in luminal sodium concentration and osmolarity along the distal convoluted tubule and collecting-duct system. First, recall that because more sodium chloride than water was reabsorbed in the loop, both the ion concentrations and osmolarity of the fluid entering the distal convoluted tubule are well below those of plasma.

Table 6-5   Summary of Major Mechanisms for Chloride Reabsorption Along the Tubule

---

Proximal: Paracellular diffusion in mid-to-late portions; driving force is high luminal chloride concentration caused by water reabsorption

Thick ascending loop: Secondary active via $Na, K, 2Cl$ cotransporter in luminal membrane

Distal convoluted tubule: (1) Paracellular diffusion; driving force is lumen-negative PD
(2) Secondary active via Na, Cl cotransporter in luminal membrane

Cortical collecting duct: (1) Paracellular diffusion; driving force is lumen-negative PD
(2) Secondary active via HCO_3^-, Cl cotransporter in luminal membrane (sodium-independent)

(The difference is less for osmolarity than for sodium because, as described in Chap. 4, another major solute—urea—is added in the loop.) As fluid flows through the distal convoluted tubule, sodium chloride reabsorption proceeds, but virtually no water is reabsorbed, despite the large osmotic gradient, because of the epithelium's low water permeability. The result is some further lowering of the luminal osmolarity.

The next tubular segment, the connecting tubule, behaves very much like the distal convoluted tubule, but events are very different beyond this segment because the water permeability of the cortical and medullary collecting ducts is subject to physiological regulation. If their water permeability is very great, the cortical collecting ducts reabsorb so much water that the luminal fluid once more equilibrates with the plasma in the cortical peritubular capillaries surrounding them, i.e., becomes isoosmotic (300 mosmol/L). After equilibrium has occurred, this segment behaves analogously to the proximal tubule, reabsorbing approximately equivalent amounts of solute and water. In contrast, when water permeability is low, the hypoosmotic fluid entering the cortical collecting duct may become even more hypoosmotic as it flows along the tubule and sodium chloride reabsorption continues, unaccompanied by equivalent water reabsorption.

The water permeability of the medullary collecting ducts shows the same variability as that of the cortical collecting ducts. Thus, in the presence of low permeability, the highly dilute fluid delivered from the cortical collecting ducts remains dilute as it flows through the medullary collecting ducts. In contrast, when the water permeability of the collecting ducts is very great, the isoosmotic fluid leaving the cortical collecting ducts is progressively concentrated in its passage through the medullary collecting ducts. (This last fact should come as a surprise since, on the basis of what has been so far described, one ought to conclude that the fluid would merely remain isoosmotic. The explanation will be given in the next section.)

The major determinant of water permeability in the collecting ducts is the posterior pituitary hormone known as **vasopressin, or antidiuretic hormone (ADH).** The first name, vasopressin, denotes the fact that this hormone can constrict arterioles and thereby increase the arterial blood pressure. The second name describes the effect of the hormone's major renal action—antidiuresis, i.e., against a high urine volume. In the absence of ADH the water permeability of the collecting ducts is very low, and little if any water is reabsorbed from these segments. Thus, most of the originally filtered water reaching the collecting ducts remains in the tubule to be excreted as a large volume of urine. On the other hand, in the presence of maximum amounts of ADH, the water permeability of the collecting ducts is very great, and the final urine volume is small—less than 1 percent of the total filtered water. Of course, the tubular response to ADH is not all-or-none but shows graded increases as the plasma concentration of ADH is increased over a certain range, thus permitting fine adjustments of water permeability and excretion.

Recall that there are two major cell types in the collecting ducts—principal cells and intercalated cells. ADH acts on the more abundant of these types, the principal cells. The principal-cell plasma membrane whose water permeability is increased in response to ADH is the luminal membrane, which is rate-limiting for water movement across the entire cell because its water permeability is so much lower than that of the basolateral membrane. (Why the luminal membrane, in contrast to almost all other plasma membranes, has such a low water permeability in the absence of ADH is not known.)

The receptors[6] for ADH are in the basolateral membrane, and the binding of ADH by its receptors results in the activation of adenylate cyclase, which catalyzes the intracellular production of cyclic AMP. This second messenger then induces, by a sequence of events, the migration of intracellular particle aggregates to the luminal membrane and the insertion into the membrane of protein channels through which water can diffuse. In the absence of ADH, these channels are withdrawn from the luminal membrane by endocytosis.

Interestingly, ADH indirectly exerts a local negative-feedback influence over its own effect. It induces the intramedullary synthesis and release of prostaglandins, which then oppose the action of ADH by interfering with ADH-induced generation of cyclic AMP. Accordingly, abnormal prostaglandin synthesis (either too much or too little) may account for the altered tubular responsiveness to ADH seen in certain

---

[6] The receptors acted on in the collecting duct are V_2 receptors. V_1 receptors on vascular smooth muscle mediate the vasoconstrictor effects of ADH.

renal diseases or during therapy with drugs that block prostaglandin synthesis.[7]

It should now be easy to understand how the kidneys produce a hypoosmotic urine, i.e., a final urine having a lower osmolarity than plasma; this occurs whenever water reabsorption lags behind solute reabsorption, i.e., when plasma ADH is reduced, and is known as **water diuresis**. In this regard, it is worth reemphasizing that even when virtually no water reabsorption occurs beyond the loop of Henle because of the absence of ADH, the reabsorption of sodium is not retarded to any great extent.[8] Therefore, intraluminal sodium concentration can be lowered almost to zero in these tubular segments.

Now a very important point: Recall that the proximal tubule behaves very differently when its water reabsorption is blocked, not by lack of ADH, which does not act proximally, but by an osmotic diuretic. Under such conditions, net sodium reabsorption is also greatly reduced because of the passive paracellular back-leak of sodium from interstitium to lumen. In the distal convoluted tubule and collecting-duct system, unlike the proximal tubule, sodium reabsorption can continue normally in the absence of water reabsorption because these segments are so much less permeable to sodium; i.e., passive paracellular fluxes are very low compared with the rate of active transcellular reabsorption. Accordingly, in comparison with the "leaky" proximal tubule, extremely large transtubular gradients for sodium can be achieved by active reabsorption in these "tight" distal segments.

Now let us return to the problem of how it is possible for the kidneys to produce a hyperosmotic urine, i.e., a urine having an osmolarity greater than that of plasma. For this to occur, water reabsorption must "get ahead" of solute reabsorption, but how can this happen if water reabsorption is always secondary to reabsorption of solute, particularly salt? The answer is given in the next section.

URINE CONCENTRATION: THE MEDULLARY COUNTERCURRENT SYSTEM

The ability of the kidneys to produce concentrated urine is not merely an academic problem. It is a major determinant of one's ability to survive without water. The human kidney can produce a maximal urinary con-

---

[7] Factors other than prostaglandins also influence cell responsiveness to ADH. For example, adrenal steroids also interfere in a variety of ways with ADH's action; therefore, patients with adrenal insufficiency manifest a tendency toward hyperresponsiveness to ADH. This partially explains why such patients reabsorb excessive amounts of water. (See Schreir and Linas in Suggested Readings.)

[8] In some species, ADH, in addition to its action on water permeability of the collecting ducts, also stimulates sodium chloride reabsorption by the thick ascending loop of Henle. This action probably does not occur in humans and so we disregard it in the text. (See Greger in Suggested Readings.)

centration of 1400 mosmol/L, almost five times the osmolarity of plasma. The sum of the urea, sulfate, phosphate, other waste products, and small number of nonwaste ions excreted each day normally averages approximately 600 mosmol. Therefore, the minimal volume of water in which this mass of solute can be dissolved equals

$$\frac{600 \text{ mosmol/day}}{1400 \text{ mosmol/L}} = 0.43 \text{ L/day}$$

This volume of urine is known as the **obligatory water loss.** It is not a fixed volume, however, but changes with different physiological states. For example, increased tissue catabolism, as during fasting or trauma, releases much solute and so increases obligatory water loss.

The obligatory water loss contributes to dehydration when a person is deprived of water intake. If we could produce a urine with an osmolarity of 6000 mosmol/L, the obligatory water loss would only be 100 mL of water, and survival time would be greatly expanded. A desert rodent, the kangaroo rat, does just that. This animal never even drinks water because the water produced by oxidation is ample for its needs.

Countercurrent Multiplication

To repeat, urinary concentration takes place as the tubular fluid flows through the medullary collecting ducts coursing toward the renal pelvis. The new fact is that the medullary interstitial fluid surrounding these ducts is very hyperosmotic. It is this interstitial hyperosmolarity that in the presence of ADH causes water to diffuse out of the medullary collecting ducts into the interstitial fluid and thence into the medullary blood vessels. The key question for urinary concentration is therefore this: How does the medullary interstitial fluid become hyperosmotic?

The complex process that sets up this interstitial hyperosmolarity is called the **countercurrent multiplier system** and takes place in those loops of Henle that, like the collecting ducts, extend into the medulla. Let us once more look at the characteristics of the loops, but this time show how water reabsorption occurs from them and the medullary interstitial fluid becomes hyperosmotic.

1 As stated earlier in this chapter, the descending limb of the loop does not reabsorb either chloride or sodium but does reabsorb water (we shall see how in a moment). Not mentioned before is that this tubular segment has a very great permeability to water but is much less permeable to the ions.

2 As described in Chap. 1, the ascending limb of the loop is not a structurally homogenous segment. It is very thin from the bend in the loop up to the outer medulla (only long loops have this thin ascending portion), where it becomes much thicker. This structural difference reflects functional differences as well. However, for simplicity, we initially present the physiological characteristics of the thick portion as though they apply to the entire ascending limb; afterward, the necessary qualifications will be made. As stated earlier in this chapter the thick ascending limb actively reabsorbs sodium and chloride via the Na,K,2Cl cotransporter, but because it is always quite impermeable to water, it does not reabsorb water.

Keeping these characteristics in mind, and assuming that the entire ascending limb has the characteristics of the thick segment, imagine the loop of Henle filled with a stationary column of fluid supplied by the proximal tubule. At first, the concentration everywhere would be 300 mosmol/L since fluid leaving the proximal tubule is isoosmotic to plasma.

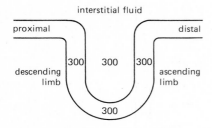

Now let the pumps in the ascending limb cause the active reabsorptive transport of sodium chloride into the interstitium until a limiting gradient (say, 200 mosmol/L) is established between ascending-limb fluid and interstitium.

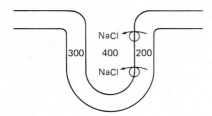

A limiting gradient is reached because the ascending limb is relatively permeable to sodium and chloride. Accordingly, passive paracellular back-flux into the lumen will ultimately counterbalance active outflux, and a steady-state limiting gradient is established.

Given the great permeability of the descending limb to water, there is a net diffusion of water[9] out of the descending limb and into the inter-

---

[9] The descending limb is not completely impermeable to sodium and chloride. Accordingly, some of these ions diffuse into the loop simultaneously with water movement out of the loop. For simplicity, we shall ignore this additional complexity. (See deRoufignac and Jamison in Suggested Readings.)

stitum until the osmolarities are equal. Therefore, water reabsorption by the *descending* limb is driven by sodium chloride reabsorption by the *ascending* limb. (Thus, as promised earlier, the generalization that water reabsorption is always secondary to solute reabsorption remains true.) The interstitial osmolarity is maintained at 400 mosmol/L during this equilibration because of continued sodium chloride transport out of the ascending limb. Note that the osmolarities of the descending limb and interstitium are equal and both are higher than that of the ascending limb.

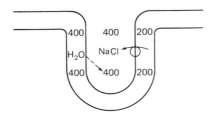

So far we have held the fluid stationary in the loop, but of course, it is actually continuously flowing. Let us look at what occurs under conditions of flow (Fig. 6-6), simplifying the analysis by assuming that flow and ion pumping occur in discontinuous, out-of-phase steps. Think of it as a series of freeze-frames in a movie. During the stationary phase, as described above, sodium chloride is transported out of the ascending limb to establish a gradient of 200 mosmol/L, and water diffuses out of the descending limb until descending limb and interstitium have the same osmolarity. During the flow phase, fluid leaves the loop via the distal convoluted tubule, and new fluid enters the loop from the proximal tubule. Also, there is nothing special about the numbers we have chosen for this illustration; i.e., there is nothing you know that could allow you to deduce these specific numbers.

Note that the intratubular fluid is progressively concentrated as it flows down the descending limb and that the medullary interstitial fluid is progressively concentrated to the same degree. Although a gradient of only 200 mosmol/L is maintained across the ascending limb at any given *horizontal level* in the medulla, there is a much larger osmotic gradient from the top of the medulla to the bottom (312 mosmol/L versus 700 mosmol/L). In other words, the gradient of 200 mosmol/L established by active ion transport has been *multiplied* because of the *countercurrent flow* (i.e., flow in opposing directions through the two limbs of a loop) within the loop. It should be emphasized that the active-ion-transport mechanism within the ascending limb is the essential component of the entire system; without it, the countercurrent flow would have no effect whatsoever on concentrations.

Now we have our concentrated interstitial fluid, but we must follow the fluid once more from the loop through the distal convoluted tubule

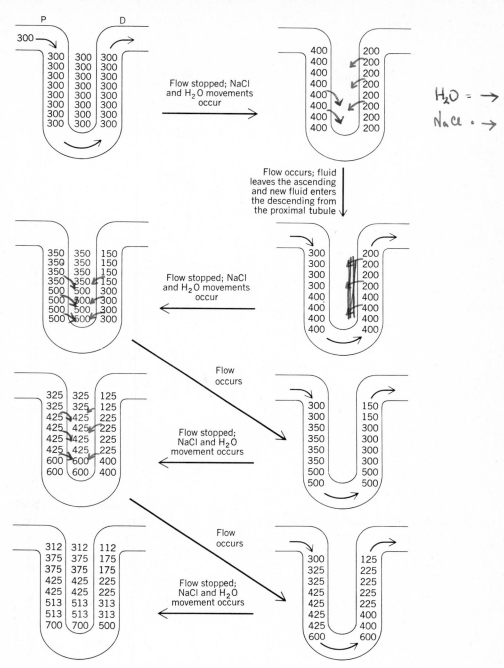

Figure 6-6 Countercurrent multiplier system in loop of Henle. *(Redrawn from RF Pitts, Physiology of the Kidney and Body Fluids, ed. 3 Chicago, Year Book 1974.)*

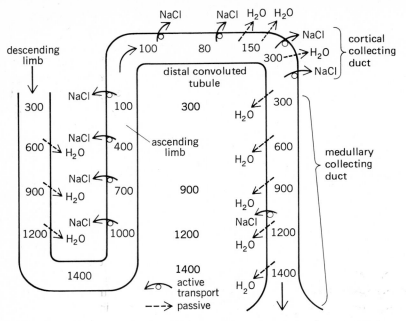

Figure 6-7 Interactions of loop of Henle and collecting duct in formation of a concentrated urine. ADH increases water permeability of the collecting ducts, both cortical and medullary. Note that interstitial osmolarity at every level is identical to descending-limb and collecting-duct osmolarity. As described in the text, this figure is oversimplified in that it assumes active transport of sodium chloride by the entire ascending loop and ignores the role of urea.

and collecting-duct system (Fig. 6-7). The countercurrent multiplier system concentrated the descending-loop fluid but then it immediately re-diluted it so that the fluid entering the distal convoluted tubule is actually more dilute than the plasma. Now we simply review the material previously presented in this chapter on the distal convoluted tubule and collecting-duct system but with the new fact that the medullary interstitium is hyperosmotic.

ADH does not act on the distal convoluted tubule or connecting tubule, and so tubular fluid remains hypoosmotic throughout these segments. ADH does act on the collecting ducts, and in its presence, water leaves the cortical collecting duct so that the tubular fluid becomes isoosmotic to cortical plasma (300 mosmol/L) by the end of this segment. Then, as the fluid flows through the medullary collecting ducts, water diffuses out of the ducts because of the hyperosmolarity of the medullary interstitium, as maintained by the loop countercurrent multiplier system. By the end of the medullary collecting duct, the tubular fluid has reached essentially the same osmolarity as the interstitiuim (maximal = 1400 mosmol/L).

This is the essence of the system: The loop countercurrent multiplier causes the interstitial fluid of the medulla to become concentrated, and it is this hyperosmolarity that in the presence of adequate ADH, will draw water out of the medullary collecting ducts and concentrate the urine. In humans, the value reached at the tip of the papilla is 1400 mosmol/L, and this is why the maximal osmolarity of the final urine is 1400 mosmol/L.

Because the osmolarity of the urine becomes greater than that of plasma only in the medullary collecting ducts, it is easy to forget that ADH acts not only on this segment but on the cortical collecting ducts as well. The action on this later segment is also important because by permitting the reabsorption there of a relatively large quantity of fluid, it ensures the delivery to the medullary collecting ducts of a volume of isoosmotic fluid small enough for efficient concentrating.

In contrast, in the presence of low plasma-ADH concentrations, the collecting ducts become relatively impermeable to water. Therefore, fluid in the cortical collecting ducts does not reequilibrate with cortical plasma, and even more important, the high interstitial osmolarity set up by the loops in the medulla is ineffective in inducing water movement out of the medullary collecting ducts. As a result, a large volume of hypoosmotic urine is excreted.

Let us summarize the overall net movement of sodium chloride and water out of the tubules and into the medullary interstitium during formation of a concentrated urine. First, sodium chloride is lost from the ascending limb by active transport of sodium and chloride.[10] This sodium chloride causes net diffusion of water out of the descending limb and the collecting ducts. In the steady state, this sodium chloride and water entering the medullary interstitium must be taken by up capillaries and carried away. This is, of course, the final step during reabsorption of fluid anywhere in the tubules, and it occurs as a result of the usual hydraulic and oncotic forces acting across the capillary wall.

As noted, the above description of the countercurrent multiplier system ignored the fact that the thin ascending loop of Henle may function differently from the thick ascending loop, specifically that it probably does not *actively* reabsorb sodium and chloride (the evidence for or against this is presently not decisive). Should this prove to be the case, what is the mechanism by which sodium chloride leaves the thin ascending limb? (That sodium chloride *does* move from the lumen of the thin ascending limb into the interstitium is well established; the question at hand here deals only with what the force is that causes these ions to move.) Several hypotheses other than active transport have been postulated, but none of them alone can presently explain all the data; they generally invoke a special role for urea, and the interested reader should consult the articles by deRoufignac and Jamison, Kokko, and Roy and Jamison cited in the Suggested Readings.

---

[10] As described earlier, sodium and chloride are also actively reabsorbed from the collecting ducts. This phenomenon helps to reduce the amount of salt lost to the urine. But it has been ignored in our analysis because it is not an important component of the countercurrent system. (But see Kokko in Suggested Readings.)

The Role of Urea in Maximizing Urine Concentration

Regardless of whether urea is somehow involved in the movement of sodium chloride out of the ascending thin limb, it is definitely involved in another way in the urine-concentrating mechanism, specifically in determining the maximal osmolarity of the urine. From the description of the countercurrent multiplier system given thus far, one would logically assume that all the solutes in the medullary interstitial fluid are sodium and chloride. Such is not the case, for approximately half of the medullary osmolarity consists of urea. However, this should not really be surprising when you recall from Chap. 4 how urea is handled beyond the loop of Henle. Luminal urea concentration rises progressively along the cortical collecting ducts and the outer medullary collecting ducts as water is reabsorbed but urea is not because these tubular segments are impermeable to it. This high urea concentration then drives diffusion out of the inner medullary collecting ducts, which are highly permeable to urea (a permeability increased by ADH). The simultaneous movement of water out of the inner medullary collecting ducts maintains a high urea concentration even as urea is being lost from these ducts.

The net result is that the urea concentration of the inner medullary interstitial fluid comes to approximate the urea concentration of the luminal fluid within adjacent medullary collecting ducts. In essence, then, urea within the tubule is balanced by urea within the interstitium. Therefore, the sodium and chloride within the interstitium need balance only the solutes *other than* urea in the tubular fluid. Thus, typical values for the case in which a highly concentrated urine is being formed are shown in Table 6-6. Note that if there were no urea in the interstitial fluid, the interstitial osmolarity caused by sodium and chloride would have to be 1400 rather than 750; i.e., more sodium chloride would have to be transported by the ascending loop of Henle.

In this description, it is easy to lose track of an essential point: Urea, unlike the sodium and chloride reabsorbed out of the ascending loop of Henle, does *not* cause water to move from tubular lumen to medullary interstitium. It balances itself but does not cause concentration of any other solute.[11]

Countercurrent Exchange: Vasa Recta

There is a unique characteristic of the medullary circulation without which the entire system could not operate, namely, the hairpin-loop anatomy of certain of the medullary vessels of the **vasa recta,** which run parallel to the loops of Henle and medullary collecting ducts. The problem is this: What would happen to the medullary gradient if the medulla were

[11] For another view, however, see Roy and Jamison, and deRoufignac and Jamison, in Suggested Readings.

Table 6-6   Composition of Medullary Interstitial Fluid and Urine During Formation of a Concentrated Urine

Interstitial fluid at tip of medulla (mosmol/L)	Urine (mosmol/L)
Urea = 650 Na+ + Cl− = 750*	Urea = 700 Nonurea solutes = 700 (Na+, Cl−, K+, urate, creatinine, etc.)

* Some other ions (e.g., potassium) contribute, to a small degree, to this osmolarity.

supplied only with ordinary capillaries? As plasma having the usual os-molarity of 300 mosmol/L entered the highly concentrated environment of the medulla, there would be massive net diffusion of sodium chloride into the capillaries and of water out of them. Thus, the interstitial gradient would soon be lost. But with hairpin loops, the sequence of events shown in Fig. 6-8 occurs. Blood enters the vessel loop at an osmolarity of 300 mosmol/L, and as it flows down the capillary loop deeper and deeper into the medulla, sodium chloride does indeed diffuse into, and water out of, the vessel. However, after the bend in the loop is reached, the blood then flows up the ascending vessel loop, where the process is almost completely reversed.

Thus, the vessel loop is acting as a so-called **countercurrent ex-changer,** which prevents the gradient from being dissipated. Note that the vessel is, itself, completely passive; i.e., it is not *creating* the medullary gradient, only protecting it. Its passive nature explains why it is called an exchanger; compare its function to that of the loop of Henle, which actively creates the gradient and is, therefore, a multiplier.

Finally, it should be noted that the hairpin-loop structure of the blood vessels minimizes losses of solute or water from the interstitium by *diffusion*. It does not, though, prevent the *bulk-flow* of medullary inter-stitial fluid into the capillaries secondary to the usual Starling forces. By this bulk-flow process, both the salt and water entering the interstitium, in equivalent amounts, from the loops and collecting ducts are carried away, and the steady-state gradient is maintained.

Clinical Changes in Urinary Concentrating Ability

A point of considerable clinical importance is that inability to achieve maximal urinary concentration occurs early in any renal disease because of interference with the establishment of the medullary gradient. Any significant change in renal structure, particulary in the medulla, can upset the intricate geometric relationships requiried for maximal countercurrent

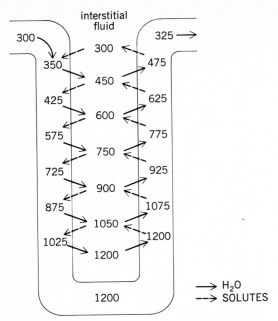

Figure 6-8 Vasa recta as countercurrent exchangers. All movements of water and solutes shown are by diffusion. Not shown is the simultaneously occurring uptake of interstitial fluid by bulk-flow. (*Redrawn from RF Pitts,* Physiology of the Kidney and Body Fluid, *ed. 3 Chicago, Year Book, 1974.*)

functioning. A change in renal blood flow to the medulla, either too much or too little, will reduce the gradient by carrying away too much or too little water and/or solute. Destruction of the loops will also reduce the gradient, as will decreased sodium and chloride pumping by the ascending limb. The latter may be caused by tubular disease or by a marked reduction in GFR and, thereby, a reduction in the supply of sodium and chloride to the loop. Another important factor is flow rate through the loop; any large increase (as, for example, in osmotic diuresis) literally "washes out" the gradient, thereby preventing concentration of the final urine. Anything that decreases maxmimal urinary concentrating ability, of course, causes an increase in obligatory water loss.

     Finally, it should be emphasized that although the entire discussion of renal concentrating ability has been in terms of urine osmolarity, a common clinical measurement of urine "concentration" is *specific gravity*. The determination of specific gravity requires only a hydrometer and is easy and cheap to perform. However, specific gravity is really a measure of urine *density*, not of concentration. Frequently, the two correlate well, but under certain circumstances they can be quite divergent since specific gravity is influenced by the nature as well as by the number of solute particles. For example, protein in the urine causes the specific gravity to be increased with little change in osmolarity.

SUMMARY
Figures 6-9 and 6-10 summarize the previously described changes in sodium, volume, and osmolarity of the tubular fluid as it flows along the nephron.

1 Approximately 65 percent of the filtered water and sodium chloride are reabsorbed in the proximal tubule, but the fluid remains isoosmotic.

2 In the loop, water is reabsorbed from the descending limb, but much more sodium chloride is reabsorbed from the ascending limb so that hypoosmotic fluid enters the distal convoluted tubule.

3 Fluid remains hypoosmotic in the distal convoluted tubule and connecting tubule with little or no water reabsorption occurring. Thus, the ascending loop of Henle, distal convoluted tubule, and connecting tubule are often referred to as *diluting segments*.

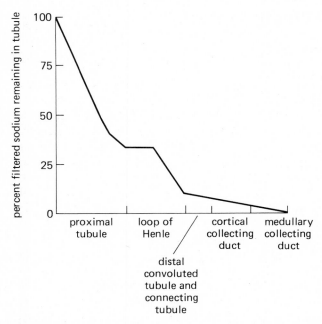

Figure 6-9 Reabsorption of sodium along the tubule. Numbers in the figure indicate the percentage of filtered sodium still remaining in the tubule at each point. Accordingly, the difference between any successive numbers indicates the percentage of filtered sodium reabsorbed by that segment. *(Courtesy Jurgen Schnermann.)*

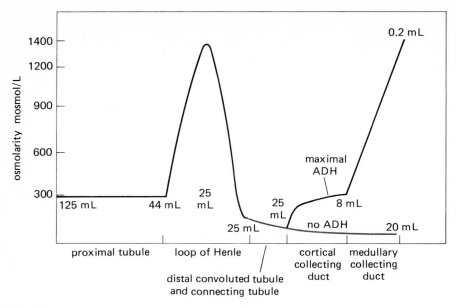

Figure 6-10 *Changes in volume and osmolarity of the tubular fluid as it flows along the nephron.*

4 Only in the collecting ducts does the presence or absence of ADH matter. With essentially no ADH, very little water is reabsorbed from the collecting ducts and these segments therefore also contribute to dilution of the urine. Consequently, a large volume of dilute urine is formed.

5 With maximal ADH, water reabsorption is high in the collecting ducts. By the end of the cortical collecting ducts, the fluid has once more become isoosmotic to cortical plasma. Almost all the remaining water is reabsorbed in the medullary collecting ducts, and a tiny volume of highly concentrated urine is formed.

6 Because of the focus on sodium chloride in this chapter, the reader may be surprised to discover that a maximally concentrated urine (1400 mosmol/L) may, under certain conditions, contain virtually no sodium chloride; the solute may be urea, creatinine, uric acid, potassium, etc. In other words, although sodium chloride *in the medullary inter-stitium* is the essential requirement for pulling water out of the medullary collecting ducts and concentrating the urine, there need be no sodium chloride in the urine itself.

Several other points of great importance should be reemphasized: (1) Excretion of large quantities of sodium *always* results in the excretion of large quantities of water. This follows from the passive nature of water reabsorption since water can be reabsorbed only if sodium is reabsorbed first. As we shall see, this relationship has considerable importance for the regulation of extracellular volume. (2) In contrast, large quantities of water can be excreted even though the urine is virtually free of sodium since a decreased ADH will increase water excretion without altering sodium transport significantly. This process we shall find crucial for the renal regulation of extracellular osmolarity.

Given the basic renal processes for handling sodium, chloride, and water, we now turn to the mechanisms by which they are controlled to regulate salt and water balance homeostatically.

Study Questions 34 to 43

7

CONTROL OF SODIUM AND WATER EXCRETION: Regulation of Plasma Volume and Osmolarity

OBJECTIVES

The student understands the renal regulation of extracellular volume and osmolarity.

1 States the formula relating filtration, reabsorption, and excretion of sodium
2 Describes the nature and locations of receptors in sodium-regulating reflexes
3 Lists the efferent inputs controlling GFR and how these inputs change as a result of changes in sodium balance or fluid volumes
4 Defines glomerulotubular balance and describes its significance
5 States the origin of aldosterone, its renal sites of action, and its effect on sodium reabsorption
6 Lists the factors controlling aldosterone secretion and states which is most important
7 Describes how intrarenal physical factors influence sodium reabsorption; states how changes in filtration fraction influence sodium reabsorption; predicts the changes in physical factors that occur with changes in sodium or fluid balance and how they alter sodium and water reabsorption.
8 States all direct and indirect effects of catecholamines and angiotensin II on sodium reabsorption
9 States the origin of atrial natriuretic factor, the stimulus for its secretion, and its effects on renal function
10 Lists all the factors that regulate sodium excretion
11 Distinguishes between primary and secondary hyperaldosteronism; describes the hormonal changes in each and the presence or absence of "escape"
12 Describes the origin of ADH and the two major reflex controls of its secretion; defines diabetes insipidus; states the effects of ADH on arterioles
13 Distinguishes between the reflex changes that occur when an individual has suffered isoosmotic fluid loss because of diarrhea as opposed to a pure-water loss, i.e., solute-water loss as opposed to pure-water loss
14 Describes the control of thirst

15 Diagrams in flow-sheet form the pathways by which sodium and water excretion are altered in response to sweating, diarrhea, hemorrhage, high- or low-salt diet

16 Lists all the actions of angiotensin II that increase fluid retention and arterial blood pressure

In normal persons, urinary sodium excretion is reflexly increased when there is a sodium excess in the body and reflexly decreased when there is a sodium deficit. These reflexes are so precise that total-body sodium normally varies by only a small percentage despite a wide range of sodium intakes and the sporadic occurrence of large losses via the skin or gastrointestinal tract.

Since sodium is freely filterable at the renal corpuscle and reabsorbed but not secreted by the tubules, the amount of sodium excreted in the final urine represents the results of two processes, glomerular filtration and tubular reabsorption:

$$\text{Sodium excretion} = \text{sodium filtered} - \text{sodium reabsorbed}$$
$$= (\text{GFR} \times P_{Na}) - \text{sodium reabsorbed}$$

It is possible, therefore, to adjust sodium excretion reflexly by controlling any of three variables: P_{Na}, GFR, sodium reabsorption.

P_{Na} may change considerably in several pathological conditions, and these changes can influence sodium excretion by altering the filtered load of sodium. However, under most physiological situations, P_{Na} changes very little (except to increase transiently after a sodium-rich meal or to decrease transiently after a large quantity of fluid containing no sodium is drunk) and may be disregarded as an important control point for regulation of sodium excretion. Accordingly, control is exerted mainly on the other two variables—GFR and sodium reabsorption.

The reflexes that control GFR and sodium reabsorption are initiated largely by baroreceptors, such as the carotid sinus, that participate in the reflexes that maintain cardiovascular pressures relatively constant. The reason that regulation of cardiovascular pressures by baroreceptors simultaneously achieves regulation of total-body sodium is that these variables are closely correlated. The chain linking total-body sodium to cardiovascular pressures is shown in Fig. 7-1: (1) Changes in total-body sodium result in similar changes in extracellular volume since sodium is essentially an extracellular solute; (2) since extracellular volume comprises plasma volume and interstitial volume, plasma volume also changes in the same direction as total-body sodium; (3) plasma volume, as a major component of total blood volume, is a major determinant of cardiovascular pressures. Thus low total-body sodium causes low cardiovascular pressures, which, via baroreceptors, initiate reflexes—decreased GFR and increased sodium reabsorption—that decrease so-

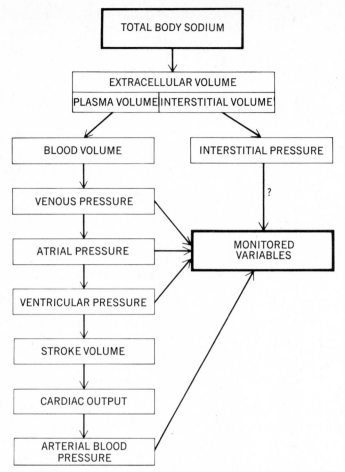

Figure 7-1   Flow sheet demonstrating the series of derivative variables dependent on total body sodium. In no case is any block in the sequence totally dependent on the previous one, for other factors are also involved. The major aim of the figure is to demonstrate how a change in body sodium will normally result in changes in a group of monitored variables that can be detected by receptors and initiate the responses controlling sodium excretion.

dium excretion, thereby retaining sodium in the body. Increases in total-body sodium have the reverse reflex effects.

The reader may be surprised that no mention has been made of receptors that monitor plasma sodium concentration. Such receptors do exist but are relatively unimportant, compared with the baroreceptors, in controlling sodium excretion.

Several qualifications should be added to this general scheme. First, this entire description has been in terms of "reflexes," but the fact is, as we shall see, several of the receptors cited are within the kidneys themselves, and no "reflex" input to or output from the kidneys is required in the sequences of events they elicit. Second, the kidneys are influenced directly by changes in the blood perfusing them—for example, by oncotic pressure—so that such nonreflex inputs related to altered sodium balance are also important in determining sodium excretion.

CONTROL OF GFR

The control of GFR has already been described, first in Chap. 2, which dealt with the factors directly determining GFR, and then in Chap. 5, which dealt with the neuroendocrine regulation of these factors. Accordingly, this section is simply a review of the salient features of those descriptions in the specific context of reflexes regulating sodium and water excretion.

Physiological Regulation of Glomerular-Capillary Pressure

Let us take a specific example: What change in GFR occurs as a result of severe salt and water loss because of diarrhea (Fig. 7-2)? The decreased plasma volume resulting from salt and water loss prevents adequate venous return, thereby reducing, in order, atrial pressure, ventricular filling, stroke volume, cardiac output, and arterial blood pressure. The fall in arterial blood pressure decreases filtration rate by lowering glomerular-capillary hydraulic pressure. Recall, however, that because of renal autoregulation arterial-pressure changes per se have only small effects on GFR over the usual physiological range.

However, the drops in blood pressure are also detected by the carotid sinuses and aortic arch, as well as by other baroreceptors in the veins and atria. The information—decreased firing rate of the baroreceptors—is relayed to the medullary cardiovascular centers, which respond by inhibiting parasympathetic outflow to the heart and by stimulating sympathetic outflow to the heart and to arteriolar smooth muscle. The sympathetic stimulation of the renal arterioles, both by the renal nerves and by epinephrine form the adrenal medulla, increases constriction of the renal arterioles. The vasoconstriction of the afferent arterioles increases the resistance to blood flow from the renal artery to the glomerular capillaries, lowering the capillary blood pressure and GFR. (As described in Chap. 5, increased sympathetic activity also causes some efferent-arteriolar constriction, which tends to increase glomerular-capillary hydraulic pressure, but the afferent effect usually predominates.)

By this mechanism, the amount of sodium filtered and, hence, the amount of sodium excreted are reduced, and further loss from the body is prevented. Conversely, an increased GFR can result reflexly from greater plasma volume and contribute to increased renal sodium loss, which returns extracellular volume to normal.

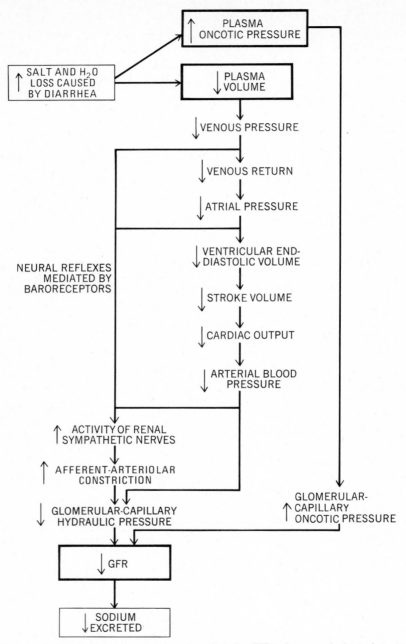

Figure 7-2 *Several major pathways by which the GFR is decreased when plasma volume decreases. The baroreceptors that initiate the sympathetic reflex are probably located in large veins and in the walls of the heart, as well as in the carotid sinuses and aortic arch. For clarity, circulating catecholamines and the renin-angiotensin system, both of which lower GFR, have not been included in the figure (see text).*

In this discussion we have emphasized the significance of the sympathetic nervous system as a major efferent pathway for GFR regulation. As described in Chap. 5, under the conditions of our example, renin secretion would also be stimulated, so that increased plasma angiotensin II would contribute to renal vasoconstriction. Since angiotensin II has such a potent effect on the efferent arteriole, its vasoconstrictor effect produces little change in GFR (but see below for its effect on K_f).

Physiological Changes in Plasma Protein Concentration

There are frequent situations in which changes in plasma volume are associated with changes in plasma protein concentration. In such situations, changes in glomerular-capillary oncotic pressure may also play an important role in the physiological raising or lowering of GFR. For example, the severe fluid loss of sweating or diarrhea (Fig. 7-2) not only will lower the plasma volume but also, because little protein is lost in the fluid, will concentrate plasma protein. The resulting increase in oncotic pressure will reduce net filtration pressure in the glomeruli and, thereby, GFR. Conversely, a marked increase in salt intake will increase plasma volume and, at least transiently, lower plasma protein concentration. The result is lowered oncotic pressure and increased GFR.

In each of these examples, the change in arterial-plasma protein concentration is in the appropriate direction to reestablish salt balance by decreasing or increasing salt excretion. Is this also true for hemorrhage? The answer is *no*. Hemorrhage per se does not immediately alter plasma protein concentration since all blood components are lost in equivalent proportions. However, the blood loss is followed by a net movement of interstitial fluid into the vascular compartment. This entry of protein-free fluid lowers the arterial-plasma protein concentration, which tends to raise GFR—an inappropriate response since sodium conservation, not increased sodium loss, is the "desired" response to hemorrhage. However, GFR does decrease in response to hemorrhage despite the fact that oncotic pressure is going in the wrong direction. Why? The answer is that decreased arterial pressure and reflexly increased sympathetic outflow to the afferent arterioles cause glomerular-capillary pressure to fall by a larger amount than oncotic pressure falls. This example is presented as a reminder of the fact that the GFR response to any given situation represents the algebraic sum of multiple forces.

Physiological Control of Glomerular
Filtration Coefficient (K_f)

In Chap. 2, it was described how, at any given net filtration pressure, GFR is proportional to the glomerular filtration coefficient (K_f). Angiotensin II, which is elevated reflexly when plasma volume is decreased, lowers K_f, by causing mesangial cells to contract, and this action contributes to the GFR-lowering effects of this hormone.

CONTROL OF TUBULAR SODIUM REABSORPTION
As far as long-term regulation of sodium excretion is concerned, the control of tubular sodium reabsorption is more important than that of GFR (even though, as we shall see, the former is somewhat dependent on the latter). For example, patients with chronic marked reductions of GFR usually maintain normal sodium excretion by decreasing tubular sodium reabsorption.

Glomerulotubular Balance
One reason that changes in the filtered load of sodium are of less importance in altering sodium excretion is the fact that the absolute reabsorption of fluid in the proximal tubules varies directly with glomerular filtration rate. This phenomenon is known as **glomerulotubular balance**. (Recall that one of the likely mechanisms for GFR autoregulation is known as *tubuloglomerular feedback*, a name unfortunately very easy to confuse with the totally different phenomenon of glomerulotubular balance being described here.) For example, if GFR is experimentally decreased by 25 percent by tightening a clamp around the renal artery, the *absolute* rate of proximal fluid reabsorption (in millimols/min) decreases by almost the same percentage. Another way of saying this is that the *percentage* of the filtrate reabsorbed proximally remains approximately constant at around 65 percent. The mechanisms responsible for adjusting tubular reabsorption to GFR are not clear.[1]

It is certain, however, that the mechanisms are completely intrarenal; i.e., glomerulotubular balance requires no external neural or hormonal input and can be shown to occur in a completely isolated kidney. The net effect of this phenomenon is to *blunt* the ability of GFR changes per se to produce *large* changes in sodium excretion.

For several reasons, however, it is incorrect to assume that because of glomerulotubular balance, sodium excretion is *completely* unaffected by changes in GFR. First, even if glomerulotubular balance were perfect, i.e., if the changes in GFR and absolute sodium reabsorption were exactly proportional, the absolute amounts of sodium leaving the proximal tubule would still change slightly when GFR changes. This can be seen in the example given in Table 7-1; in this example, even though reabsorption stays fixed at 66.7 percent, the absolute amount of sodium leaving the

---

[1] Part of the explanation is simply that when GFR is altered, there is an altered supply of substances cotransported with sodium—glucose, amino acids, etc.—to later portions of the proximal tubule.

Table 7-1   Effect of "Perfect" Glomerulotubular Balance on the Mass of
Sodium Leaving the Proximal Tubule

GFR, L/min	P_{Na}, mmol/L	Filtered mmol/min	Reabsorbed proximally (66.7% of filtered), mmol/min	Leaving proximal, mmol/min
0.124	145	18	12	6
0.165	145	24	16	8
0.062	145	9	6	3

proximal tubule rises when GFR is increased and falls when GFR is decreased. Second, glomerulotubular balance is not really perfect; i.e., the changes in GFR and reabsorption are not usually exactly proportional. Thus, the proper conclusion is that changes in the filtered load of sodium per se *do* result in changes in sodium excretion, but the changes are greatly mitigated by glomerulotubular balance.

Glomerulotubular balance is really a second line of defense preventing changes in hemodynamics per se from causing large changes in sodium excretion. The first line of defense is autoregulation of GFR. In other words, GFR autoregulation prevents GFR from changing too much in direct response to changes in blood pressure, and glomerulotubular balance blunts the sodium-excretion response to whatever GFR change does occur. Glomerulotubular balance allows major responsibility for homeostatic control of sodium excretion to reside in those factors (to be described next) that act, independently of GFR changes, to influence tubular reabsorption of sodium.

We also see here another analogy between autoregulation and glomerulotubular balance in that both are manifest in their "pure" forms only when the kidneys are manipulated in relative isolation from the rest of the body, as by altering renal perfusion through the use of renal-artery clamps. In contrast, when GFR is made to change by doing something to the whole animal or person, say by infusing large quantities of isotonic saline, glomerulotubular balance is overridden by other inputs to the kidney so that the proximal tubule is observed to reabsorb a smaller percentage (in our saline infusion example) or a larger percentage (in situations like severe hemorrhage) than usual. Thus, like autoregulation, glomerulotubular balance merely dampens the change in sodium excretion "desired" for the particular physiological situation. For example, during hemorrhage, sodium excretion decreases—the desired homeostatic effect—but glomerulotubular balance and autoregulation both cause the decrease to be less than if these two phenomena did not exist.

Aldosterone

The single most important controller of sodium reabsorption is **aldosterone**, the hormone produced by the **adrenal cortex**, specifically in the cortical area known as the **zona glomerulosa**. (This last term is somewhat unfortunate because it sounds like a description of a kidney area rather than of an adrenal zone.)

Aldosterone stimulates sodium reabsorption by the connecting tubule and the cortical collecting duct. Because the cortical collecting duct is by far the more important site, for simplicity we will deal only with it. The cell type in the cortical collecting duct acted on by aldosterone is the **principal cell**, the same cell acted on by ADH. An action on this late portion of the nephron is just what one would expect for a fine-tuning input since more than 90 percent of the filtered sodium has already been reabsorbed—by the proximal tubule, ascending loop of Henle, and distal convoluted tubule—by the time the collecting-duct system is reached.

The total quantity of sodium reabsorption dependent on the influence of aldosterone is approximately 2 percent of the total filtered sodium. Thus, all other factors remaining constant, in the complete absence of aldosterone one would excrete 2 percent of the filtered sodium, whereas in the presence of maximal plasma concentrations of aldosterone, virtually no sodium would be excreted. Two percent of the filtered sodium may, at first thought, seem small, but it is actually very large because of the huge volume of glomerular filtrate:

$$
\begin{aligned}
\text{Total filtered NaCl/day} &= \text{GFR} \times P_{Na} \\
&= 180 \text{ L/day} \times 145 \text{ mmol/L} \\
&= 26{,}100 \text{ mmol/day}
\end{aligned}
$$

Thus, aldosterone controls the reabsorption of $0.02 \times 26{,}100$ mmol/day $= 522$ mmol/day. In terms of sodium chloride, the form in which most sodium is ingested, this amounts to approximately 30 g NaCl per day, an amount considerably more than the average person eats. Therefore, by reflex variation of plasma concentrations of aldosterone between minimal and maximal, the excretion of sodium can be finely adjusted to the intake so that total-body sodium and extracellular volume remain constant.

It is interesting that aldosterone also stimulates sodium transport by other epithelia in the body, namely, by sweat and salivary ducts and by the intestine. The net effect is the same as that exerted on the kidney—movement of sodium from lumen to blood. Thus, aldosterone is an all-purpose stimulator of sodium retention.

Aldosterone exerts its effect by combining with intracellular receptors and stimulating, in the nucleus, synthesis of mRNA, which then mediates translation of specific proteins. At least one of the newly synthesized proteins somehow opens previously closed sodium channels in the luminal membrane. This in turn allows greater entry of sodium into the cell, increased cell sodium concentration, and increased pumping of sodium across the basolateral membrane by Na,K-ATPase pumps. In this schema, the increased pumping across the basolateral membrane is driven

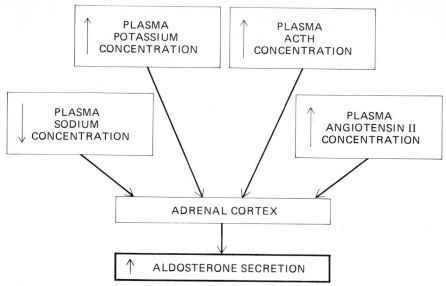

Figure 7-3 Direct controls of aldosterone secretion. A reversal of all arrows in the top boxes would lead to a decrease in aldosterone secretion.

simply by the increased cell sodium concentration. Over a longer span of time, an increase in the synthesis of the Na,K-ATPase pumps also occurs.

Because aldosterone's enhancement of sodium reabsorption requires time (at least 45 min) for protein synthesis, decreases in sodium excretion that occur within minutes (as, for example, immediately upon standing up) are clearly not caused by increased aldosterone.

Control of Aldosterone Secretion   How is aldosterone secretion controlled? At least four distinct direct inputs to the adrenal gland are recognized at present (Fig. 7-3): (1) plasma sodium concentration, (2) plasma potassium concentration, (3) adrenocorticotropic hormone (ACTH), and (4) angiotensin II.

The first two of these inputs are not mediated by nerves or by hormones. Rather, the adrenal cortex responds to the sodium and potassium concentrations of the blood perfusing it. This is one of the true "sodium" receptors referred to earlier in this chapter, and the fact that aldosterone secretion is controlled, in part, by plasma sodium concentration makes good sense: Increased plasma sodium → decreased aldosterone secretion → decreased tubular sodium reabsorption → increased sodium excretion → decreased plasma sodium concentration. However, in humans, this is a very minor control of aldosterone secretion—a fact that also makes sense teleologically since plasma sodium *concentration* generally changes very little despite marked changes in extracellular *volume*. Water movements into or out of body cells tend to keep osmolarity and, thereby, plasma sodium concentration relatively stable. In contrast, the influence of plasma potassium concentration on aldosterone secretion is important and will be described in the chapter on renal handling of potassium.

   ACTH is the hormone from the anterior pituitary that controls secretion of the other major adrenocortical hormone, cortisol. There is no question that when ACTH is secreted in very large amounts, as during physical trauma, it also stimulates aldosterone secretion. Moreover, even in lower concentrations, ACTH is permissive for other stimulators of aldosterone secretion. Thus, ACTH does play significant roles in the control of aldosterone secretion. However, the secretion of ACTH is not keyed to sodium homeostasis; i.e., it does not usually participate in reflexes specifically "aimed" at maintaining a constant level of body sodium.

   We are left with our fourth input, angiotensin II, as the most important known controller of aldosterone secretion in sodium-regulating reflexes.[2] As described in Chap. 1, the primary determinant of the plasma concentration of angiotensin II is the plasma concentration of renin, which is itself determined mainly by the rate of renin secretion. Accordingly, control of aldosterone secretion is in large part ultimately determined by those factors that regulate renin secretion (at this point, the reader should review the section on control of renin secretion in Chap. 5). Thus, when plasma volume is reduced by hemorrhage, diarrhea, etc., renin secretion is stimulated, which leads, via angiotensin II, to an increased aldosterone secretion (Fig. 7-4).

Factors Other Than Aldosterone Influencing Tubular Reabsorption of Sodium

Despite its unquestioned primary importance in the regulation of tubular reabsorption of sodium, aldosterone is not the only factor that does so in response to alterations in body-sodium balance. Identification of these other factors has been the most investigated subject in renal physiology during the past two decades, but we are still left with uncertainty concerning the quantitative significance of the many such factors that have been uncovered.

   Intrarenal Physical Factors: Interstitial Hydraulic Pressure   Recall from the previous chapter that renal interstitial hydraulic pressure is one of the forces driving the last step in fluid reabsorption—movement into the

[2] There is also evidence for the probable existence of other controllers of aldosterone secretion in addition to the four well-established ones given in the text. Dopamine and atrial natriuretic hormone inhibit aldosterone secretion, whereas several pituitary hormones—β-endorphin, β-lipotropin, and a protein termed aldosterone-stimulating hormone—stimulate it. (See Carey and Sen in Suggested Readings.)

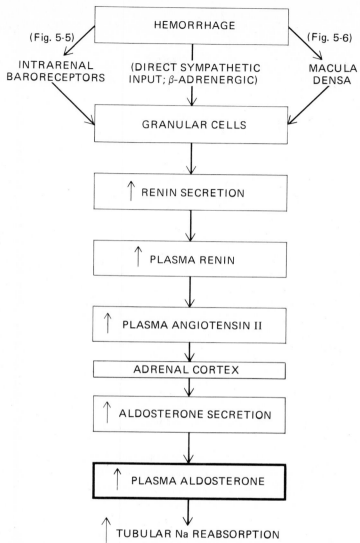

Figure 7-4 Pathway by which aldosterone secretion is increased during hemorrhage.

peritubular capillaries. One might logically, but wrongly, conclude, there-fore, that increased renal interstitial pressure would favor reabsorption. The observed fact, however, is that whenever renal interstitial pressure is *elevated*, there is a tendency for sodium reabsorption to be *decreased*. Similarly, decreased renal interstitial pressure tends to cause increased sodium reabsorption. These relationships hold mainly for the proximal tubule. The mechanism is not known but may involve leakage of sodium, which had been actively transported across the tubular cells into the interstitium, across the tight junctions and back into the tubular lumen. Whatever the mechanism, renal interstitial pressure is one of the determinants of net sodium reabsorption, the relationship being an inverse one.

The two factors that are most important in setting the steady-state interstitial hydraulic pressure in the kidneys are really the same as in any other location in the body—the capillary hydraulic pressure and the plasma oncotic pressure—since these are the dominant forces determining the steady-state volume of fluid in the interstitium. Increased hydraulic pressure inside the capillary tends to raise interstitial hydraulic pressure by causing fluid to accumulate in the interstitium; a decrease in plasma oncotic pressure does precisely the same. Therefore, via its effects on interstitial hydraulic pressure, increased hydraulic pressure in the peritubular capillaries reduces tubular sodium reabsorption. Conversely, decreased peritubular-capillary hydraulic pressure facilitates reabsorption. Increased oncotic pressure in peritubular-capillary plasma also facilitates reabsorption, whereas decreased oncotic pressure reduces reabsorption.

Thus, earlier in this chapter we saw that changes in *glomerular-capillary* hydraulic and oncotic pressures were controlled to regulate GFR and, thereby, sodium excretion; now we see that analogous changes in the *peritubular-capillary* hydraulic and oncotic pressures help regulate sodium reabsorption and, thereby, sodium excretion.

Teleologically, it makes good sense that such changes in these so-called **intrarenal physical factors** regulate sodium balance and plasma volume by altering sodium reabsorption. Volume depletion, as in our example of diarrhea, causes decreased peritubular-capillary hydraulic pressure, just as it does decreased glomerular-capillary hydraulic pressure, because of reduced arterial pressure and reflex renal vasoconstriction (Fig. 7-5).[3] The effect of the reduced pressure is to enhance sodium reabsorption. The volume depletion caused by the diarrhea also causes concentration of plasma protein, and this increased plasma oncotic pressure also enhances tubular sodium reabsorption, just as it reduces GFR.

In the last example, the change in peritubular-capillary oncotic pressure simply reflects a change in systemic plasma oncotic pressure. Now, we introduce a new but predictable fact: Peritubular-capillary oncotic pressure can be changed independently of any changes in systemic oncotic pressure. The information needed to understand this phenomenon has already been given: Peritubular-capillary oncotic pressure *always* differs from systemic oncotic pressure since the plasma proteins are concentrated by loss of protein-free filtrate during passage through the glomerular capillaries. The degree of oncotic-pressure increase depends on the fraction of the renal plasma flow that is filtered at the glomerulus;

---

[3] The decreased venous pressure that occurs in volume depletion also contributes to the decrease in peritubular-capillary pressure.

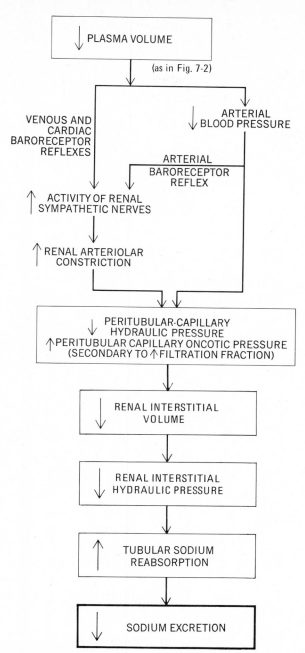

Figure 7-5 Pathway by which changes in intrarenal physical factors are elicited by changes in plasma volume. Compare this figure with Fig. 7-2, the figure for GFR control; the same inputs that tend to lower GFR also tend to increase sodium reabsorption via changes in intrarenal physical factors. As with Fig. 7-2, for simplicity, circulating catecholamines and the renin-angiotensin system, both of which have similar effects on intrarenal physical factors, have not been included.

this **filtration fraction** is not always the same but varies depending on the distribution of renal arteriolar constriction. Recall from Chap. 5 that reflex vasoconstriction mediated either by the renal nerves or by circulating agents generally affects not only the afferent arterioles but the efferent arterioles as well. The net result is that both GFR and RPF decrease but the latter more than the former; therefore, the filtration fraction, GFR/RPF, increases. Accordingly, there occurs a larger than normal increase in oncotic pressure along the peritubular capillaries and increased reabsorption of sodium (Fig. 7-5).

The examples used thus far in this section were for situations in which changes in intrarenal physical factors *favor* sodium reabsorption. However, intrarenal physical factors can also change in the direction that decreases sodium reabsorption. The most prominent example is the phenomenon called **pressure natriuresis**, the increase in sodium excretion caused by increased renal arterial pressure, which raises renal interstitial hydraulic pressure.[4]

Direct Tubular Effects of Renal Nerves   Preceding sections have detailed how the renal sympathetic nerves can influence sodium reabsorption by altering not only renin secretion but also intrarenal physical factors. In addition, the renal nerves also stimulate sodium reabsorption by *direct* action on the tubular cells themselves. The proximal tubule[5] is the major site affected by this direct input, which has the same adaptive significance as the indirect renal effects of altered sympathetic activity.

Thus, the increased renal sympathetic nerve activity triggered via the extarenal baroreceptor reflexes (or other signals such as fright) leads by a variety of mechanisms, summarized in Table 7-2, to decreased sodium excretion.

Direct Tubular Effects of Angiotensin II   As we have seen, angiotensin II enhances sodium reabsorption indirectly both through its stimulation of aldosterone and, because it constricts renal arterioles and raises filtration fraction, through its effects on intrarenal physical factors. In addition, like the renal nerves, it acts directly on the renal cells themselves to stimulate sodium reabsorption.[6] Again, as in the case with the renal nerves, the proximal tubule is the major segment affected by this direct response.

---

[4] However, increased renal interstitial pressure is almost certainly not the only factor that contributes to pressure natriureseis. (See Knox and Granger in Suggested Readings.)

[5] The receptors involved are alpha$_1$-adrenergic, the same type that mediates vasoconstriction by arterioles. There are also alpha$_2$-adrenergic receptors in various tubular segments, and experimental activation of these by infused catecholamines can inhibit sodium and water reabsorption; their physiological significance is not known. (See Pettinger et al. and Quinn.)

[6] A source of potential confusion is the fact that angiotensin II, when present in extremely high ("pharmacological") amounts, inhibits sodium reabsorption rather than stimulating it.

Table 7-2 Effects of Renal Nerve Stimulation*

1. Increases renin secretion via direct action on beta$_1$-adrenergic receptors.
2. Increases sodium reabsorption via direct action on tubular cells (alpha$_1$-adrenergic receptors).
3. Increases renal arteriolar vasoconstriction (alpha$_1$-adenergic receptors), leading to decreased GFR, decreased RBF, and increased filtration fraction. These lead, indirectly, as described in the text, to increased renin secretion and increased sodium reabsorption.

* These effects are listed in the order in which they are elicited as the frequency of renal nerve impulses is increased to higher and higher values. Note that the direct effects on both renin secretion and sodium reabsorption occur at lower stimulation levels than those required to elicit vasoconstriction.

Atrial Natriuretic Factor (ANF) and Hypothalamic Natriuretic Factor Many of the cells in the cardiac atria secrete a peptide hormone called **atrial natriuretic factor (ANF)**; other commonly used names for this hormone include atrial natriuretic peptide, atriopeptin, and auriculin. ANF produces an increase in urinary sodium excretion, in part by increasing GFR[7] but also by acting directly on the tubule (mainly the medullary collecting duct) to inhibit sodium reabsorption. In addition, ANF can inhibit renin secretion and angiotensin-induced aldosterone secretion, actions that contribute indirectly to decreased sodium reabsorption and increased sodium excretion.

The major stimulus for increased secretion of ANF is distention of the atria, which occurs during plasma volume expansion. This is probably the stimulus for the increased ANF that occurs in persons on a high-salt diet. Although it is generally assumed that ANF plays a physiological role in the regulation of sodium excretion in this and other situations, it is not presently possible to quantitate its contribution.

ANF is not the only substance suspected of functioning as a physiological natriuretic hormone. Hypothalamic extracts contain a low-molecular-weight substance that can inhibit Na,K-ATPase in the renal tubules (and other tissues), and this substance has been found in the blood in some situations associated with expansion of plasma fluid volume. Whether it really participates in the normal regulation of sodium excretion, however, is unknown.

Other Known Humoral Agents Cortisol, estrogen, growth hormone, and insulin are all known to enhance sodium reabsorption,[8] whereas glucagon, progesterone, and parathyroid hormone all decrease it. When the level of any of these hormones is elevated (as, for example, estrogen

---

[7] ANF increases GFR by relaxing glomerular mesangial cells (K_f) and by dilating the afferent arteriole. Indeed, it is a general relaxer of vascular smooth muscle, and it is possible that the major function of ANF is to regulate blood pressure and blood flow rather than renal function. (See articles by Blaine and by Goetz in Suggested Readings.)

[8] In some species, but probably not human, ADH also stimulates sodium reabsorption, specifically by the thick ascending loop (see Greger in Suggested Readings for Chap. 6).

during pregnancy), it will exert a significant influence on sodium reabsorption and, thereby, excretion. However, the secretion of these hormones, unlike the factors described in the previous paragraph, are not reflexly controlled specifically to regulate sodium balance homeostatically.[9]

Also of great interest is the possible role played by intrarenal humoral systems, particularly the prostaglandins, the kinins, and dopamine. These agents are known to be able to reduce sodium reabsorption by altering intrarenal physical factors (as we have seen, they are all vasodilators) and/or by direct actions on the tubular cells. Their concentrations are also known to change with alterations of sodium balance, but it is not yet possible to integrate these systems with any assurance into the overall picture of renal sodium regulation.

SUMMARY OF THE CONTROL OF SODIUM EXCRETION

The control of sodium excretion depends mainly on the control of two variables of renal function, the GFR and the rate of sodium reabsorption (Table 7-3). The latter is controlled most importantly by the renin-angiotensin-aldosterone hormone system but also by the sympathetic nervous system and other less well-defined factors, including intrarenal physical factors and atrial natriuretic factor. There is great flexibility in such a multifactorial system. Thus, for example, although the renal sympathetic nerves influence GFR, renin secretion, intrarenal physical factors, and the reabsorptive activity of the tubular cells, a transplanted and, therefore, denervated kidney maintains sodium homeostasis quite well because of the many other known (and unknown) nonneural factors involved. Overall, the one input whose absence causes the greatest difficulty in sodium regulation is aldosterone (but see below).

The reflexes that control both GFR and sodium reabsorption are essentially blood-pressure-regulating reflexes since they are most frequently initiated by changes in cardiovascular pressures acting via baroreceptors. This is fitting, as described earlier, since cardiovascular function depends on an adequate plasma volume, which, as a component of the extracellular fluid volume, normally reflects the mass of sodium in the body. In normal persons, these regulatory mechanisms are so precise that sodium balance does not vary by more than a small percentage despite marked changes in dietary intake or losses caused by sweating, vomiting, diarrhea, hemorrhage, or burns.

---

[9] Parathyroid hormone may be an exception to this generalization. Although its secretion is controlled mainly by plasma calcium, it is also increased during volume expansion and may contribute to the inhibition of proximal-tubular sodium reabsorption in this situation (see Seldin and Giebisch in Suggested Readings).

Table 7-3   Changes in These Factors Influence Sodium Excretion
in Response to Changes in Plasma Volume

Filtration of Sodium
 GFR
 Plasma sodium concentration (of minor importance except in severe disorders)

Tubular reabsorption of sodium
 GFR (glomerlotubular balance)
 Aldosterone
 Intrarenal physical factors
 Renal nerves (direct tubular effects)
 Angiotensin II (direct tubular effects)
 Atrial natriuretic factor
 ? Hypothalamic natriuretic factor
 ? Prostaglandins, kinins, and dopamine

Abnormal Sodium Retention

In several types of disease, however, sodium balance becomes deranged by the failure of the kidneys to excrete sodium normally. Sodium excretion may fall virtually to zero and remain there despite continued sodium ingestion, and the person retains large quantities of sodium and water, leading to the abnormal expansion of extracellular fluid and formation of edema. An important example of this phenomenon is **congestive heart failure**. A patient with a failing heart (i.e., a heart whose contractility is too low to maintain the cardiac output required for the body's metabolic requirements) usually manifests decreased GFR and increased activities of the renin-angiotensin-aldosterone system and renal sympathetic nerves. In addition renal filtration fraction is almost always increased—a situation that causes increased oncotic pressure in the peritubular capillaries. All these, and perhaps other as yet unidentified sodium-retaining factors, contribute to the almost complete reabsorption of sodium.[10]

Why do these sodium-retaining reflexes continue to be elicited despite the fact that the person with heart failure is in markedly positive and progressively increasing sodium balance? The answer stems from the fact, described earlier, that total extracellular volume itself is not directly monitored. In the normal person there is no discrepancy between changes in plasma volume, extracellular volume, and total-body sodium, on the one hand, and cardiovascular pressures on the other. Thus, a reflex triggered by a change in cardiovascular pressures will end up homeostatically regulating body sodium and extracellular volume. In contrast, in heart failure, there is a discontinuity between these two groups of variables; specifically, the person has a lower than normal cardiac output and

---

[10] ANF is one factor that does *not* contribute to the sodium retention of heart failure because the plasma concentration of this hormone is increased by the atrial distension and is, therefore, opposing the retention.

hence arterial pressures at any given plasma and extracellular volume. The arterial baroreceptors reduce their firing rates because of the decrease in mean and pulsatile arterial pressure,[11] and this initiates sodium-retaining reflexes just as would occur in a normal person whose cardiac output had been reduced because of hemorrhage or severe diarrhea.

There are several other conditions, specifically the liver disease **cirrhosis** and the kidney syndrome **nephrosis**, that tend to produce sodium retention of this kind. They, too, are characterized by persistent sodium-retaining reflexes (decreased GFR, increased aldosterone, etc.) despite progressive overexpansion of extracellular fluid and formation of edema, as in congestive heart failure. All these edematous conditions, including congestive heart failure, are sometimes termed diseases of **secondary hyperaldosteronism** because they are usually associated with increased secretion of aldosterone *secondary* to increased angiotensin II, which in turn is due to the inappropriate reflexes just described.

At one time it was thought that the elevated aldosterone was sufficient in itself to cause progressive accumulation of sodium. It is now recognized that such is not the case and that one or more of the other factors that influence sodium excretion must also be operating to maintain the retention. This is nicely illustrated by the difference in sodium handling between **primary hyperaldosteronism** and the diseases of secondary hyperaldosteronism. Primary hyperaldosteronism is characterized by persistent oversecretion of aldosterone because of a primary adrenal defect, usually an aldosterone-producing tumor. Because of the increased aldosterone, sodium retention does occur *initially*, but after a few days, there occurs an "escape" from the effects of aldosterone, i.e., a return to normal sodium excretion despite the continued presence of increased aldosterone. After balance is reestablished, a persistent, small positive sodium balance does remain. What has happened is that the initial sodium retention causes expansion of extracellular volume and total-body sodium, which then initiates sodium-losing responses: (1) GFR often rises; and (2) the factors (e.g., intrarenal physical factors, increased ANF, decreased renal sympathetic activity, and decreased angiotension II concentration) other than aldosterone that act on the tubule reduce sodium reabsorption. The net effect of these responses is to compensate for aldosterone-induced hyperreabsorption, and so sodium excretion is restored to normal.

In other words persistent, progressive sodium retention cannot be induced by an abnormality in only one of the factors controlling sodium excretion since reflexes will rapidly be induced whereby opposing changes in other factors will restore normal sodium excretion. Only when many inputs are altering sodium excretion, either appropriately, as in

---

[11] In addition, baroreceptors in the great veins and cardiac chambers appear to be damaged by (or adapted to) the engorgement occurring in these locations and manifest decreased rates of firing despite the marked degree of distention.

sodium depletion, or inappropriately, as in the diseases of secondary hyperaldosteronism, will sodium excretion remain continuously near zero. In these latter diseases "escape" does not occur from the effects of persistently elevated aldosterone.

A variety of drugs, collectively termed **diuretics**, are used in congestive heart failure and other situations to enhance sodium excretion by blocking sodium reabsorption. A table summarizing their mechanisms of actions is given in Appendix A and provides a nice review not only of sodium reabsorptive mechanisms but also of the interplay among the renal handling of sodium, potassium, and hydrogen-ion. If you choose to look at this table, therefore, wait until you have finished Chap. 9 to do so.

ADH SECRETION AND EXTRACELLULAR VOLUME

Although we have spoken of plasma-volume regulation only in terms of the control of sodium excretion, it is clear that to be most effective in altering plasma volume, the changes in sodium excretion must be accompanied by equivalent changes in water excretion. We have already pointed out that the ability of water to follow when sodium is reabsorbed depends on ADH. Accordingly, it is critical that decreased extracellular volume reflexly call forth increased ADH production as well as increased aldosterone secretion. What is the nature of this reflex? ADH is an octapeptide produced by a discrete group of hypothalamic neurons whose cell bodies are located in the supraoptic and paraventricular nuclei and whose axons terminate in the posterior pituitary, from which ADH is released into the blood. These hypothalamic neurons receive input from venous, cardiac, and arterial baroreceptors.[12]

The baroreceptors are stimulated by increased cardiovascular pressures, and the impulses resulting from this stimulation are transmitted via afferent nerves and ascending pathways to the hypothalamus, where they inhibit the ADH-producing cells. Conversely, decreased cardiovascular pressures cause less firing by the baroreceptors and a resulting stimulation of ADH synthesis and release. The adaptive value of these baroreceptor reflexes is to help restore extracellular volume and, hence, blood pressure (Fig. 7-6).

There is a second adaptive value to this reflex: Large decreases in plasma volume elicit, by way of the cardiovascular baroreceptors, such high concentrations of ADH—concentrations much higher than those needed to produce maximal antidiuresis—that the hormone is able to exert direct vasoconstrictor effects on arteriolar smooth muscle. The

[12] In nonprimates, baroreceptors in the left atrium are the major volume receptors controlling ADH secretion, but the picture is presently unclear for humans (see Menninger in Suggested Readings).

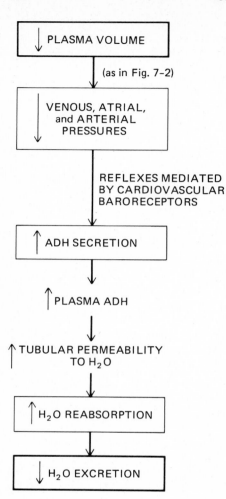

Figure 7-6 Pathway by which ADH secretion is increased when plasma volume decreases. A reversal of all arrows would show how ADH secretion is decreased and water excretion increased when plasma volume increases. In humans, it is not clear which baroreceptors are most important in this response.

result is increased total peripheral resistance, which helps raise arterial blood pressure independently of the more slowly occurring restoration of bodily fluid volumes. Also renal arterioles and mesangial cells participate in this constrictor response, and so a high plasma concentration of ADH, quite apart from its effect on tubular water permeability, may promote retention of both sodium and water by lowering GFR.

Another factor capable of stimulating ADH secretion is angiotensin II. Thus, the renin-angiotensin system may play a role in enhancing water reabsorption (via ADH) as it does sodium (via aldosterone), but the quantitative importance of this pathway is much less then that of the baroreceptor reflexes for ADH described above.[13]

Finally, it should be noted that ADH is also elevated in the diseases, like congestive heart failure, characterized by secondary hyper-aldosteronism with edema. Decreased input from the arterial barorecep-tors is the most likely cause.

ADH AND THE RENAL REGULATION OF EXTRACELLULAR OSMOLARITY

We turn now to the renal compensation for pure-water losses or gains, e.g., the situation in which a person drinks 2 L of water. No change in the total bodily salt content occurs; only the total water changes. The most efficient compensatory mechanism is for the kidneys to excrete the ex-cess water without altering their usual excretion of salt, and this is precisely what they do. ADH secretion is reflexly inhibited, as will be described below; water permeability of the collecting ducts becomes very low; sodium reabsorption proceeds normally, but water is unable to follow; and a large volume of extremely dilute urine is excreted. In this manner, the excess pure water is eliminated.

Conversely, when a pure-water deficit occurs, ADH secretion is reflexly stimulated, water permeability of the collecting ducts is in-creased, water reabsorption is maximal, the final urine volume becomes extremely small, and its osmolarity is considerably greater than that of the plasma. By this means, relatively less of the filtered water than solute is excreted—which is equivalent to adding pure water to the body—and the pure-water deficit is compensated for.

To reiterate, pure-water deficits or gains are compensated for by partially dissociating water excretion from salt excretion through changes in ADH secretion. What receptor input controls ADH under such condi-tions? The answer is changes in bodily fluid osmolarity. This makes adaptive sense since bodily fluid osmolarity, not plasma volume, is the variable most affected by pure-water gains or deficits. The osmoreceptors involved are located in the hypothalamus, the liver, and probably other sites as well; the mechanism by which they detect changes in osmolarity is unknown.[14]

[13] There is even disagreement about whether plasma concentrations of angiotensin II are ever high enough physiologically to stimulate ADH secretion (see Robertson in Sug-gested Readings).

[14] Some evidence suggests that these receptors may actually be sensitive to sodium rather than to osmolarity. The end result is the same since sodium is normally the major determinant of osmolarity. Of clinical interest is the fact that the receptors are not affected by changes in plasma urea or glucose; accordingly, the increases in these substances in uremia and diabetes mellitus, respectively, do not increase ADH secretion. (See Robertson in Suggested Readings.)

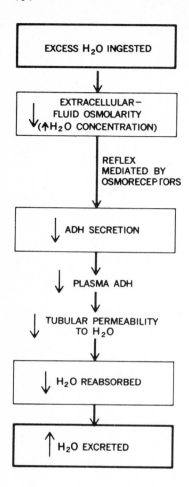

Figure 7-7 Pathway by which ADH secretion is lowered and water excretion raised when excess water is ingested.

The hypothalamic cells that secrete ADH receive neural input from these osmoreceptors. Via these connections, an increase in osmolarity stimulates them and increases their rate of ADH secretion. Conversely, decreased osmolarity inhibits ADH secretion (Fig. 7-7). The osmoreceptors are extraordinarily sensitive: For example, a 1 percent decrease in osmolarity, producible by drinking less than 500 ml of water, is enough to trigger, via the osmoreceptors, a reduction in ADH secretion adequate to increase water excretion.

We have now described two different major afferent pathways controlling the ADH-secreting hypothalamic cells, one from baroreceptors and one from osmoreceptors. These hypothalamic cells are, therefore, true integrators, whose rate of activity is determined by the total synaptic input to them. Thus, a simultaneous increase in plasma volume and decrease in bodily fluid osmolarity causes strong inhibition of ADH secretion. Conversely, the opposite changes in plasma volume and osmolarity produce very marked stimulation of ADH secretion because there seems to be a synergism between these two inputs. But what happens when baroreceptor and osmoreceptor inputs oppose each other, for example, if plasma volume and osmolarity are both decreased? In general, the osmoreceptor influence predominates over that of the baroreceptor when changes in osmolarity and plasma volume are small to moderate because of the greater sensitivity of the osmoreceptors. However, a very large change in plasma volume will take precedence over decreased bodily fluid osmolarity in influencing ADH secretion.

To add to the complexity, the ADH-secreting cells may respond, as we have seen, to angiotensin II, and they also receive synaptic input from many other brain areas. Thus, ADH secretion and, hence, urine flow can be altered by pain, fear, and a variety of other factors, including drugs such as alcohol, which inhibits ADH release. However, this complexity should not obscure the generalization that ADH secretion is determined over the long term primarily by the states of bodily fluid osmolarity and plasma volume.

The disease **diabetes insipidus**, which is different from diabetes mellitus, or sugar diabetes, illustrates what happens when the ADH system is disrupted. Diabetes insipidus is characterized by the constant excretion of a large volume of highly dilute urine, as much as 25 L/day. In most cases, the flow can be restored to normal by the administration of ADH. These patients have lost the ability to produce ADH, usually as a result of damage to the hypothalamus. Thus, collecting-duct permeability to water is low and unchanging regardless of extracellular osmolarity or volume. In contrast, other diseases are associated with inappropriately large secretion of ADH. As is predictable, patients with these diseases manifest decreased plasma osmolarity because of the excessive reabsorption of pure water.

This completes our description of the control of renal-tubular sodium and water reabsorption. Figure 7-8 summarizes many of the factors known to control these processes in response to severe sweating, as in exercise.

THIRST AND SALT APPETITE

Now we must turn to the other component of fluid balance—control of salt and water intake. It must be emphasized that large deficits of salt and water can be only partly compensated for by renal conservation and that ingestion is the ultimate compensatory mechanism.

The centers that mediate thirst are located in the hypothalamus and

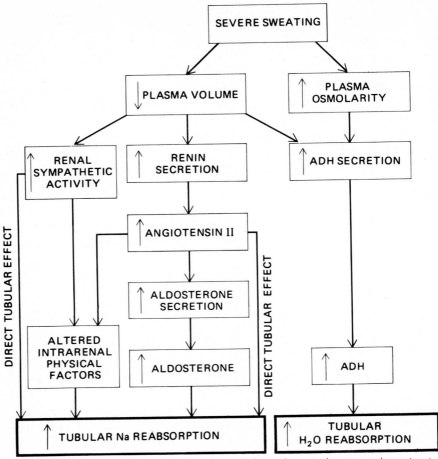

Figure 7-8 Summary of factors that increase tubular sodium and water reabsorption in severe sweating. These changes, coupled with the decrease in GFR that also occurs, homeostatically reduce urinary sodium and water loss.

are very close to those areas that produce ADH. The subjective feeling of **thirst**, which drives one to obtain and ingest water, is stimulated both by reduced plasma volume and by increased bodily fluid osmolarity. The adaptive significance of both are self-evident. Note that these are precisely the same changes that stimulate ADH production, and the receptors—osmoreceptors and cardiovascular baroreceptors—that initiate the ADH–controlling reflexes are probably identical to those that trigger thirst. The thirst response, however, is significantly less sensitive than is the ADH response.

There are also other pathways controlling thirst. For example, dryness of the mouth and throat causes profound thirst, which is relieved by merely moistening them. Also when animals such as the camel (and humans, to a lesser extent) become markedly dehydrated, they will rapidly drink just enough water to replace their previous losses and then stop. What is amazing is that when they stop, the water has not yet had time to be absorbed from the gastrointestinal tract into the blood. Some kind of metering of the water intake by the gastrointestinal tract has occurred, but its nature remains a mystery.

Angiotensin II is yet another factor that stimulates thirst—by a direct effect on the brain—and this hormone constitutes one of the pathways by which thirst is stimulated when extracellular volume is decreased.

Salt appetite, which is the analogue of thirst, is also an extremely important component of sodium homeostasis in most mammals, particularly in the herbivores. It is clear that salt appetite in these species is innate and consists of two comoponents: (1) *hedonistic* appetite and (2) *regulatory* appetite. In other words, (1) animals like salt and eat it whenever they can, regardless of whether they are salt-deficient, and (2) their drive to obtain salt is markedly increased in the presence of deficiency.

The significance of these animal studies for humans, however, is unclear. Salt craving does seem to occur in humans who are severely salt-depleted, but the contribution of such regulatory salt appetite to everyday sodium homeostasis in normal persons is probably slight. On the other hand, humans do seem to have a strong hedonistic appetite for salt, as manifested by almost universally large intakes of sodium whenever it is cheap and readily available. Thus, the average American intake of salt is 10 to 15 g/day despite the fact that humans can survive quite normally on less than 0.5 g/day. Present evidence suggests that a large salt intake may be a contributor to the pathogenesis of hypertension.

SUMMARY OF THE EFFECTS OF ANGIOTENSIN II

We have presented various effects of angiotensin II throughout this book, and this seems a good place to summarize them. Angiotensin II exerts a wide array of effects on many bodily sites, but the common denominator of those with which we are concerned is that they all favor both salt retention and elevation of arterial blood pressure. Figure 7-9 summarizes these effects, adding the fact, not previously mentioned, that angiotensin II facilitates the activity of the sympathetic nervous system. It is crucial to recognize that when renin secretion is elevated in response to *physiological* stimuli, such as sodium deprivation, all the effects of angiotensin II shown in Fig. 7-9 serve to minimize fluid depletion and to prevent blood pressure from falling below normal. In contrast, when an

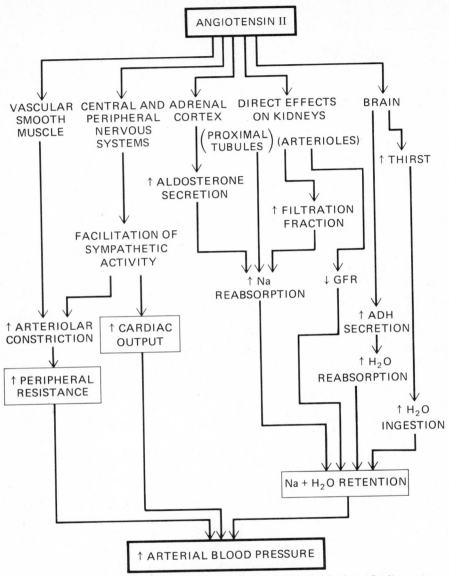

Figure 7-9 *Summary of those angiotensin-mediated actions that facilitate fluid retention and elevate the arterial blood pressure. The arrow connecting "Na and H$_2$O retention" to "arterial blood pressure" is a shortcut for the sake of simplicity—of course, fluid retention influences arterial blood pressure only by altering cardiac output and peripheral resistance.*

inappropriate increase in renin secretion occurs because of disease (as in renal-artery stenosis, for example), these effects will tend to elevate the blood pressure above normal.

Study questions: 44 to 59

8

RENAL REGULATION OF POTASSIUM BALANCE

OBJECTIVES

The student understands the internal exchanges of potassium.
1 States the normal distribution of body potassium
2 States the effects of epinephrine, insulin, aldosterone, acidosis, and alkolosis on potassium movement into cells

The student understands the renal regulation of potassium.
1 Describes the basic renal mechanisms for handling potassium in each tubular segment, including medullary cycling
2 Contrasts the contribution of each tubular segment to potassium handling during a high- and low-potassium diet
3 Describes the mechanism by which potassium secretion is accomplished by the cortical collecting duct
4 Lists the inputs that control the rate of potassium secretion by the cortical collecting duct to regulate potassium balance homeostatically
5 Describes the pathway by which changes in potassium balance influence aldosterone secretion; states aldosterone's mechanism of action
6 Describes the relationship between potassium secretion and fluid delivery to the cortical collecting duct; explains how this relationship prevents changes in aldosterone produced by altered sodium balance from perturbing potassium secretion; states the effects of most diuretics on potassium secretion; contrasts potassium secretion in persons with primary versus secondary hyper-aldosteronism
7 Describes the effects of alkalosis on potassium secretion and balance
8 Predicts the changes in potassium excretion and balance occurring in diarrhea and diabetes mellitus

The potassium concentration of the extracellular fluid is a closely regulated quantity. The importance of maintaining this concentration stems primarily from the role of potassium in the excitability of nerve and muscle. The resting membrane potentials of these tissues are directly related to the ratio of intracellular to extracellular potassium concentration. Raising the extracellular potassium concentration lowers the resting membrane potential, thus increasing cell excitability. Conversely, lowering the extracellular potassium concentration hyperpolarizes cell membranes and reduces their excitability.

Extracellular potassium concentration is a function of two variables: (1) the total amount of potassium in the body and (2) the distribution of this potassium between the extracellular and intracellular fluid compartments. The first variable, total-body potassium, is determined by the relative rates of potassium intake and excretion. Normal individuals remain in potassium balance, as they do in sodium balance, by excreting daily an amount of urinary potassium equal to the amount of potassium ingested minus the small amounts eliminated in the feces and sweat. Normally potassium losses via sweat and the gastrointestinal tract are small, although greater than sodium losses, but very large quantities can be lost from the tract during vomiting or diarrhea. Again, the control of renal function is the major mechanism by which total-body potassium is regulated.

However, before describing the renal handling of potassium, we must briefly summarize the less well-understood but very important second variable determining extracellular potassium concentration—the distribution of total-body potassium between the extracellular and intracellular fluid compartments.

REGULATION OF INTERNAL POTASSIUM DISTRIBUTION

Approximately 98 percent of total body potassium is located within cells because of the Na,K-ATPase plasma-membrane pumps, which actively transport potassium into cells. Since the amount of potassium in the extracellular compartment is so small, compared with that inside the cells, even very small shifts of potassium into or out of the cells can produce large changes in extracellular potassium concentration. Such shifts, particularly in muscle and liver, are to some extent under physiological control. Therefore, when extracellular potassium concentration changes because of changes either in total-body potassium (i.e., imbalances between intake and excretion) or internal shifts secondary to other events (cell damage, for example), potassium moves into or out of the cells, thereby minimizing the changes in extracellular concentration. The major factors involved in these homeostatic processes are epinephrine, insulin and aldosterone.

Epinephrine causes increased net movement of potassium into cells, particularly muscle. This effect is mediated by beta-adrenergic receptors, but the mechanism underlying the net movement is not known. This effect is probably of greatest importance during exercise and trauma. In these situations potassium moves out of the exercising muscle cells or the damaged cells, which raises extracellular potassium concentration. However, at the same time, exercise or trauma increases adrenomedullary secretion of epinephrine, and this hormone's stimulation of potassium uptake by other cells partially offsets the outflow from the exercising or damaged cells.

Insulin, at physiological concentrations, exerts a tonic permissive effect promoting net movement of potassium into muscle, liver, and other tissues. Moreover, a very large increase in plasma potassium concentration stimulates insulin secretion, and the additional insulin induces greater potassium uptake by the cells—a negative feedback system for opposing elevations in plasma potassium concentration.

Aldosterone also facilitates potassium movement into the cells. As we shall see, the secretion of this hormone is increased by high plasma potassium, and so its effect on cellular uptake of potassium constitutes another negative feedback mechanism for opposing elevations in plasma potassium concentration. Conversely, a decrease in aldosterone causes decreased movement of potassium into the cells.

Thus far, the discussion has dealt with factors that *homeostatically* regulate internal potassium movements to minimize changes in extracellular potassium concentration. However, other factors can influence potassium movements into or out of cells but are not homeostatic mechanisms for regulating extracellular potassium. Instead they may displace extracellular potassium concentration away from normal. The most important of these is the hydrogen-ion concentration of bodily fluids: An increase in hydrogen-ion concentration (acidosis) is often associated with net potassium movement out of cells, and alkalosis with net potassium movement into them.[1] It is as though potassium and hydrogen ions were "exchanging" across plasma membranes (i.e., hydrogen ions moving into the cell during acidosis and out during alkalosis, with potassium doing just the opposite), but the precise mechanism underlying these "exchanges" has not yet been clarified.

BASIC RENAL MECHANISMS

Potassium is freely filterable at the glomerulus.[2] The amounts of potassium excreted in the urine are usually a small fraction (10 to 15 percent) of the filtered quantity. This fact establishes the existence of tubular potassium reabsorption. However, under certain conditions excreted po-

---

[1] There are many exceptions to these generalizations. (See the article by Adrogue and Madias in Suggested Readings.)

[2] Recent evidence suggests that at least in some species, approximately 10 percent of plasma potassium may actually be protein-bound, but this is not yet generally accepted for human beings.

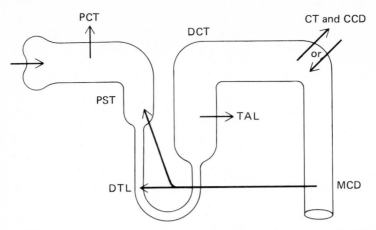

Figure 8-1 Handling of potassium by different nephron segments. Filtration occurs at the renal corpuscles, whereas all subsequent arrows denote net tubular reabsorption or secretion. See text for discussion of each segment. PCT = proximal convoluted tubule; PST = proximal straight tubule; DTL = descending thin limb; TAL = thick ascending limb; CT = connecting tubule; CCD = cortical collecting duct; MCD = medullary collecting duct.

tassium may actually exceed the filtered quantity. This fact establishes that tubular potassium secretion also exists. Thus, potassium can undergo either net tubular reabsorption or net tubular secretion.

Let us follow potassium along the length of a nephron in an individual on a normal- or high-potassium diet and in stable potassium balance (Fig. 8-1). First, potassium reabsorption occurs in the proximal convoluted tubule. It is primarily a diffusion process, the concentration gradient for which is created, as for urea, by water reabsorption.[3] By the end of the proximal convoluted tubule, approximately 50 percent of the filtered potassium has been reabsorbed.

Then in the straight portion of the proximal tubule and in the descending limb of the loop of Henle, potassium secretion occurs, mainly by diffusion down a potassium concentration gradient from interstitium to lumen. The source of this interstitial potassium will be described shortly.

In the thick ascending limb, potassium reabsorption again occurs.[4] This reabsorption is so effective that the amount of potassium entering the distal convoluted tubule is approximately 10 percent of the mass originally filtered at the glomerulus. In other words, the proximal convoluted tubule reabsorbs 50 percent of the filtered potassium, and the thick

[3] The lumen-positive potential across the later proximal tubule also drives potassium reabsorption by diffusion. In addition, some reabsorption is caused by solvent drag; i.e., potassium is "dragged" along with the reabsorbed water.

[4] This reabsorption is both passive and active. The passive component occurs paracellularly because of the lumen-positive potential, whereas the active component is driven by the Na,K,2Cl luminal cotransporter described in the section on countercurrent multiplication of sodium.

ascending limb reabsorbs another 40 percent of the filtered potassium *plus* whatever potassium had been secreted into the straight proximal tubule and descending limb.[5]

Now for the rest of the tubule, keeping in mind that we are describing the situation for a person on a normal- or high-potassium diet: The distal convoluted tubule transports little, if any, potassium, and we shall ignore it. The connecting tubule and cortical collecting duct actively secrete potassium, so that the amount in the tubule increases considerably. The greater the potassium intake the greater the amount of potassium secreted. Because the connecting tubule functions similarly to the cortical collecting duct and the latter is the most important of the two, we shall for simplicity not make further reference in the remainder of this chapter to the connecting tubule.

The final nephron segment, the medullary collecting duct, passively reabsorbs some potassium, the remainder being excreted in the urine. The potassium reabsorbed from this segment is the source of the potassium that is secreted into the straight proximal tubule and descending loop of Henle. Thus, there is a recycling of potassium from the medullary collecting ducts to the straight proximal tubules and descending loops analagous to that described for urea in Chap. 4.

The net result of all these transport processes is that most of the potassium appearing in the urine is potassium that was secreted by the cortical collecting duct.

Now let us go through the nephron again, but this time for an individual who is on a very low-potassium diet or who is potassium-depleted for some other reason, e.g., diarrhea. The proximal tubule and the ascending loop still reabsorb almost all the filtered potassium and whatever is recycling from the medullary collecting duct. The amount of potassium reaching the distal convoluted tubule, therefore, is about the same as the amount reaching it when the individual was on the normal- or high-potassium diet. Again, the distal convoluted tubule does little, if anything, to this small amount of potassium, which then enters the collecting duct system. Now the radical difference appears: *The cortical collecting duct does not secrete any potassium.* Indeed, it may actually reabsorb potassium.[6] The medullary collecting duct also reabsorbs potassium, just as it does in the person with normal- or high-potassium

---

[5] These numbers are for short-looped nephrons; the pattern is probably the same for long-looped nephrons but quantification is not available (see articles by Jacobson and by Jamison in Suggested Readings).

[6] As stated in the next section, it is the principal cells that secrete potassium. Some of the far less numerous intercalated cells of the cortical collecting duct, in contrast, actively reabsorb potassium. Normally, principal-cell secretion is much greater than intercalated-call reabsorption, and so the cortical collecting duct shows net secretion. During potassium depletion, however, the principal cells cease their secretion, and so net reabsorption occurs. (See Field and Giebisch in Suggested Readings.)

intake. The end-result is that only a very small amount of potassium is excreted.

These examples should reinforce the following important generalization: *Differences in potassium excretion over the usual physiological range are due primarily to differences in the amount of potassium secreted by the cortical collecting duct.* It is this variable that is controlled to regulate homeostatically urinary potassium excretion. There is little, if any, homeostatic control over the rest of the nephron with regard to potassium.[7]

So dominant is this secretory process that in describing the control of potassium excretion, we will tend to ignore any contribution of changes in either filtered potassium (GFR $\times P_K$) or tubular transport proximal to the collecting-duct system. It must be pointed out, however, that under certain abnormal conditions, potassium reabsorption in the proximal tubule or loop may be decreased and that a large quantity of the potassium excreted may represent filtered potassium that has not been reabsorbed. For example, diuretics that inhibit sodium reabsorption by the proximal tubule or thick ascending loop also inhibit potassium reabsorption at these sites. Another situation characterized by inhibition of proximal and loop potassium reabsorption is osmotic diuresis. Just as is true for sodium, an osmotic diuretic interferes with potassium reabsorption, and this is one reason for the marked urinary loss of potassium suffered by patients with uncontrolled diabetes mellitus.

MECHANISM OF POTASSIUM SECRETION IN THE CORTICAL COLLECTING DUCT

To restate our critical generalization: Differences in potassium excretion over the usual physiological range are due primarily to differences in the amount of potassium secreted by the cortical collecting duct. The cortical collecting duct cells that secrete potassium are the **principal cells**, the same cells we described earlier as the aldosterone-regulatable reabsorbers of sodium and also the cells affected by ADH. Figure 8-2 summarizes the pathway for potassium secretion in these cells. The critical event is the active transport of potassium from interstitial fluid across the basolateral membrane into the cell. This active transport step, which is mediated via Na,K-ATPase pumps, creates a very high intracellular potassium concentration so that there is a concentration gradient favoring net potassium diffusion from cell into lumen through the numerous luminal potassium channels in this tubular segment. (There is also some diffusion through basolateral membrane channels from the cell back into the interstitial fluid.)

---

[7] During potassium depletion there may be some regulatory stimulation of potassium reabsorption in both the cortical and medullary collecting ducts. (See Field and Giebisch in Suggested Readings.)

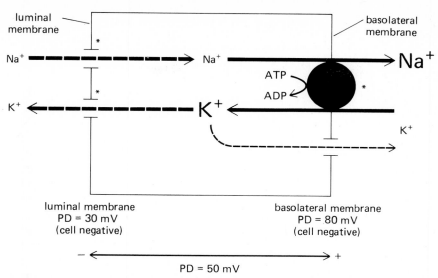

Figure 8-2 Model of transcellular sodium and potassium transport by principal cells of the cortical collecting duct. The reabsorption of sodium and secretion of potassium by these cells are regulated by aldosterone (ADH also acts on them to regulate their water permeability). The dashed lines denote net diffusional fluxes through channels. The thicknesses of the lines are not drawn to scale; that is, they serve only to emphasize which flux is greatest at each membrane, not how much greater. The asterisk (*) indicates a process controlled by aldosterone, as described in the text. Note that the model shows only transcellular potassium movement; the tight junctions between these cells, however, are not completely impermeable to potassium so that some small fraction of potassium secretion probably does occur by the paracellular route, driven by the favorable potential difference from interstitial fluid to lumen. This "transtubular" potential difference of 50 mV is merely the algebraic sum of the luminal and basolateral membrane potentials.

Note that the potassium concentration gradient across the luminal membrane is opposed by an electrical force (30mV, cell-negative) that favors net diffusion from lumen to cell. However this opposing electrical force is not as large as the chemical force (the concentration gradient), and the result is net diffusion of potassium into the lumen. Thus, secretion involves active transport of potassium into the cell across the basolateral membrane and passive exit across the luminal membrane. Clearly, in such a model, activity of the basolateral pump emerges as the dominant force driving overall active secretion.

HOMEOSTATIC CONTROL OF POTASSIUM SECRETION BY THE CORTICAL COLLECTING DUCT

What are the factors that influence potassium secretion by the principal cells of the cortical collecting duct to achieve homeostasis of bodily potassium? The single most important factor is as follows: When a high-potassium diet is ingested (Fig. 8-3), plasma potassium concentration

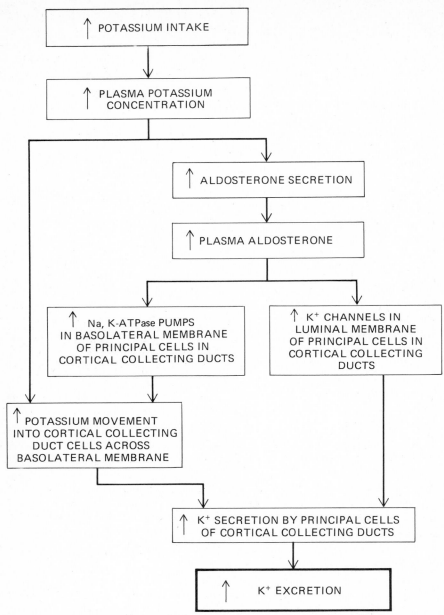

Figure 8-3 Pathways by which an increased potassium intake induces increased potassium excretion by increasing the potassium secretion of principal cells in the cortical collecting duct.

increases, even though very slightly, and this drives enhanced basolateral uptake via the basolateral Na,K-ATPase pumps. The resulting increase in intracellar potassium concentration enhances the gradient for potassium movement into the lumen and raises potassium secretion. Conversely a low-potassium diet or a negative potassium balance, e.g., from diarrhea, lowers potassium concentration in the principal cells; this reduces potassium secretion and excretion, thereby helping to reestablish potassium balance.

A second important factor linking potassium secretion to potassium balance is the hormone **aldosterone,** which besides stimulating tubular sodium reabsorption by the principal cells, simultaneously enhances tubular potassium secretion by these cells (Fig. 8-3). The reflex by which changes in plasma volume control aldosterone production is completely different from the reflex initiated by an excess or deficit of potassium. The former, as we saw in Chap. 7, constitutes a complex pathway involving renin and angiotensin II. The latter, however, is much simpler (Fig. 8-3): The aldosterone-secreting cells of the adrenal cortex are sensitive to the potassium concentration of the extracellular fluid bathing them. Increased intake of potassium leads to increased extracellular potassium concentration, which in turn directly stimulates aldosterone production by the adrenal cortex. The resulting increase in plasma aldosterone concentration stimulates potassium secretion by the cortical collecting duct and thereby eliminates the excess potassium from the body.

Conversely, lowered extracellular potassium concentration decreases aldosterone production and thereby reduces tubular potassium secretion; less potassium than usual is execreted in the urine, thus helping to restore the normal extracellular potassium concentration.

How does aldosterone increase potassium secretion (Fig. 8-3)? Recall from Chap. 7 that this hormone, in addition to increasing luminal-membrane sodium channels, causes an increase in the number of basolateral-membrane Na,K-ATPase pumps. This increases basolateral potassium transport into the cell, hence increasing intracellular potassium concentration and the gradient for movement into the lumen. Aldosterone also increases luminal-membrane permeability to potassium by increasing the number of open potassium channels in the luminal membrane, so that the enhanced gradient for diffusion is even more effective in driving luminal entry. Thus, aldosterone increases luminal-membrane permeability not only to sodium but to potassium as well (Fig. 8-2).

The examples used in this section have been concerned with changes in dietary potassium intake. However, it should be emphasized that when total-body potassium balance is perturbed by primary changes in potassium output, as for example in severe diarrhea, the same mechanisms described above operate homeostatically to control potassium secretion in the cortical collecting duct and thereby help to restore potassium balance. Thus, the potassium depletion resulting from diarrhea would

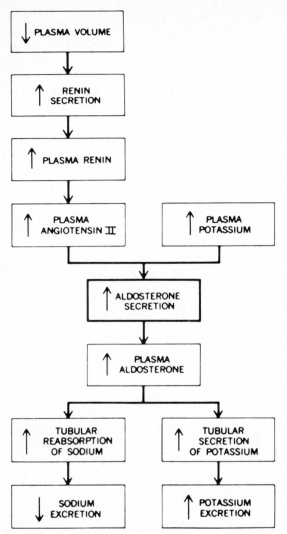

Figure 8-4 Summary of the control of aldosterone by plasma volume and plasma potassium concentration and the effects of aldosterone on renal handling of sodium and potassium. Not shown in the figure is the fact that aldosterone exerts a third effect on the tubule: It stimulates tubular hydrogen-ion secretion, as described in Chap. 9.

tend to inhibit aldosterone secretion and, hence, distal potassium secretion.

The phrase "tend to inhibit" in the last sentence highlights the fact that as we have seen, potassium is not the only regulator of aldosterone secretion (Fig. 8-4). It should be evident that a conflict will arise if decreases—as in the above example—or increases in *both* potassium and plasma volume occur simultaneously since these two changes drive aldosterone production in opposite directions. Whether aldosterone increases or decreases in such situations depends on the relative magnitu_es of the opposing inputs. In general, changes in sodium balance have greater effects on aldosterone secretion than do equivalent changes in potassium balance.

This raises a potential problem for potassium homeostasis: If aldosterone secretion is altered, via the renin-angiotensin system, because of altered *sodium* balance, will the change in plasma aldosterone cause an imbalance of body *potassium* by inducing inappropriate changes in potassium secretion? In most physiological situations the answer is no, and the explanation is given in the next section.

Potassium Secretion and Fluid Delivery to the Cortical Collecting Duct

To answer the question raised in the previous paragraph, we must first introduce what seems like an unrelated fact: An increased delivery of fluid to the cortical collecting duct causes this tubular segment to increase its secretion of potassium. The mechanism is as follows: Recall that the final step in potassium secretion—movement across the luminal membrane—is a passive process driven by the concentration gradient for potassium from cell to lumen. A large volume of flow through the cortical collecting duct, just by its diluting effect, keeps the luminal concentration low as potassium enters from the cell, and so the gradient for passive entry is maintained at a high value. Therefore, luminal entry is enhanced.

It is this relationship between fluid delivery and potassium secretion that permits changes in aldosterone caused by sodium imbalance to regulate sodium without perturbing potassium. Let us take an example (Fig. 8-5).A person on a high-sodium diet has a low plasma aldosterone concentration because of decreased renin secretion, and this will tend to decrease potassium secretion. Simultaneously, however, the person on the high-sodium diet has both increased GFR and reduced proximal sodium reabsorption (because of changes in intrarenal physical factors, low angiotensin II, and low sympathetic input), thereby increasing fluid delivery to the more distal nephron segments. The increased fluid flow through the cortical collecting duct tends to increase potassium secretion. The net result is that the effects on potassium secretion of the low aldosterone and high fluid delivery essentially counterbalance each other, and little if any change in potasium secretion and, hence, excretion occurs. Thus, the decreased aldosterone caused by increased sodium intake can increase sodium execretion without producing significant potassium retention.

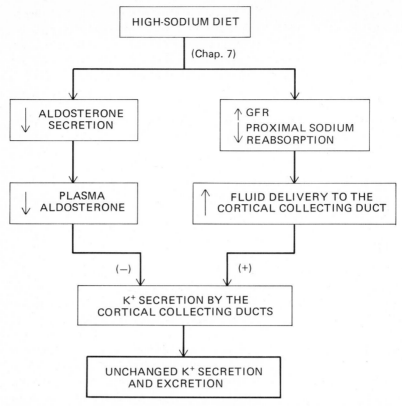

Figure 8-5 A high-sodium diet decreases plasma aldosterone (via the renin-angiotensin system) but simultaneously increases fluid delivery to the cortical collecting duct. These inputs have opposing effects on potassium secretion by the cortical collecting duct, so that little change occurs.

This same explanation, in reverse, applies to sodium-depleted persons and to persons with congestive heart failure or other diseases of secondary hyperaldosteronism (you might need to review, in Chap. 7, why renal function in these categories is similar). Such persons have high aldosterone, which will tend to increase potassium secretion, but they also have low fluid delivery to the cortical collecting duct, which will tend to reduce potassium secretion. The net effect is relatively unchanged potassium secretion and excretion.[8]

[8] Contrast this result to that in the patient with primary hyperaldosteronism. This person has both elevated aldosterone and normal or increased delivery of fluid to the cortical collecting duct (review the changes in renal sodium handling that occur in primary hyperaldosteronism—Chap. 7) and so suffers a marked and persistent elevation in potassium secretion and execretion, enough to cause serious potassium depletion.

To summarize, changes in aldosterone secretion—in either direction—caused by changes in sodium balance do not usually cause major perturbations in potassium balance. The reason is that these situations are usually associated with cortical-collecting-duct flows that oppose the effect of the altered aldosterone on potassium secretion.

Effects of Diuretics   We introduced the fact that increased fluid flow to the cortical collecting duct increases potassium secretion in the context of aldosterone and "conflicts" between sodium and potassium balance in order to stress its physiologic role. Now, however, we must emphasize that the most striking clinical manifestation of this relationship is a pathophysiological one: Potassium excretion is almost always increased in persons undergoing osmotic diuresis or treatment with diuretics that act on the proximal tubule, loop of Henle, or distal convoluted tubule. The potassium loss may cause severe potassium depletion.

The increased potassium excretion is due partly to the fact that as noted earlier in this chapter, these types of diuretics inhibit not only sodium reabsorption but also potassium reabsorption at their sites of action. However, most of the increased potassium excretion is due not to this decreased reabsorption but to increased potassium secretion by the cortical collecting duct. In all these diuretic states, the volume of fluid flowing into the collecting duct per unit time is increased by the upstream inhibition of sodium and water reabsorption, and it is this increased flow that drives increased potassium secretion and, hence, excretion (Fig. 8-6).

To reinforce this point further, let us integrate this information with that of the previous section on aldosterone. As stated there, the elevated aldosterone in persons with heart failure or other diseases of secondary hyperaldosteronism generally does not cause potassium hypersecretion because these people simultaneously have low fluid delivery to the cortical collecting duct. But what happens when such persons are treated with diuretics to eliminate their retained sodium and water? The diuretics increase fluid delivery to the cortical collecting duct, and now the person has both increased aldosterone and increased flow to the cortical collecting duct. This combination tends to cause marked increases in potassium secretion and excretion. To avoid this combination, drugs that block the renal actions of aldosterone may be given; such drugs are diuretic because they block aldosterone's stimulation of sodium reabsorption, but unlike other diuretics, they are "potassium-sparing" because they simultaneously block aldosterone's stimulation of potassium secretion. (See Appendix A for a description of another class of diuretics that does not increase potassium secretion.)

Finally, it should be noted that the *water diuresis* that accompanies low plasma ADH, unlike the diuretic situations described in the previous

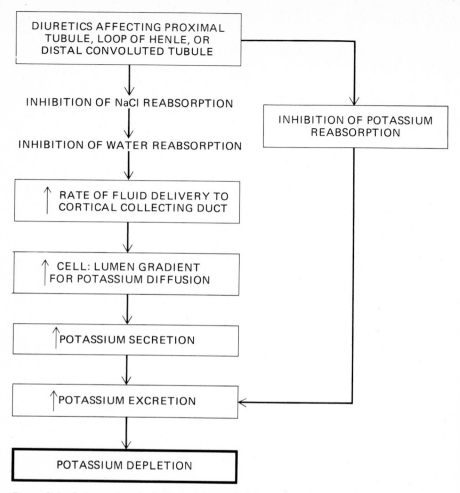

```
┌─────────────────────────────┐                    ┌──────────────────────────┐
│  DIURETICS AFFECTING PROXIMAL│                    │                          │
│  TUBULE, LOOP OF HENLE, OR   │───────────────┐    │                          │
│  DISTAL CONVOLUTED TUBULE    │               │    │                          │
└─────────────────────────────┘               │    │                          │
              │                                │    │  INHIBITION OF POTASSIUM │
              ▼                                └───▶│  REABSORPTION            │
   INHIBITION OF NaCl REABSORPTION                  │                          │
              │                                     └──────────────────────────┘
              ▼                                               │
   INHIBITION OF WATER REABSORPTION                           │
              │                                               │
              ▼                                               │
┌─────────────────────────────┐                              │
│ ↑ RATE OF FLUID DELIVERY TO  │                              │
│   CORTICAL COLLECTING DUCT   │                              │
└─────────────────────────────┘                              │
              │                                               │
              ▼                                               │
┌─────────────────────────────┐                              │
│ ↑ CELL: LUMEN GRADIENT       │                              │
│   FOR POTASSIUM DIFFUSION    │                              │
└─────────────────────────────┘                              │
              │                                               │
              ▼                                               │
┌─────────────────────────────┐                              │
│ ↑POTASSIUM SECRETION         │                              │
└─────────────────────────────┘                              │
              │                                               │
              ▼                                               │
┌─────────────────────────────┐                              │
│ ↑POTASSIUM EXCRETION         │◀─────────────────────────────┘
└─────────────────────────────┘
              │
              ▼
┌─────────────────────────────┐
│   POTASSIUM DEPLETION        │
└─────────────────────────────┘
```

Figure 8-6 Pathway by which diuretic drugs affecting the proximal tubule, loop of Henle, or distal convoluted tubule cause potassium depletion. The decrease in potassium reabsorption is a less important factor than is the increased secretion in causing the increased potassium excretion.

section, is *not* associated with increased potassium secretion. The reasons are not completely understood.[9]

[9] In all the other diuretic situations described in the previous section, the increased volume flow through the cortical collecting duct is caused by increased delivery of fluid from more proximal segments. In contrast low ADH—water diuresis—does not increase delivery of fluid *to* this segment. Nevertheless, water diuresis is associated with increased flow *through* the cortical collecting duct because water reabsorption by this segment is reduced by the absence of ADH and so more water remains in the cortical collecting duct. This increased flow should, therefore, cause increased secretion and excretion of potassium. But as stated in the text, this does not occur. One possible explanation is that ADH itself may directly stimulate potassium secretion. Accordingly, there would be counterbalancing effects during water diuresis: (1) Increased flow causes increased potassium secretion, but (2) the absence of ADH's direct effect causes decreased potassium secretion. The net result would be virtually no change in potassium secretion. (See Field and Giebisch in Suggested Readings.)

THE EFFECTS OF ACID-BASE CHANGES ON POTASSIUM SECRETION

The last section explained how primary changes in sodium balance do not usually perturb potassium balance. Now we shall see that such is *not* the case for primary changes in hydrogen-ion balance. Indeed, primary acid-base disturbances are a major cause of secondary potassium imbalance because they cause marked changes in potassium secretion and excretion.

The most important empirical finding is as follows: The existence of an alkalosis, either metabolic or respiratory in origin, induces increased potassium secretion and excretion (Fig. 8-7). Thus, a patient suffering from metabolic alkalosis (induced, say, by vomiting) will manifest increased urinary excretion of potassium solely as a result of the alkalosis and will, therefore, become potassium-deficient.

The stimulatory effects of alkalosis on potassium secretion are mediated, at least in part, through an increase in the potassium concentration of principal cells in the cortical collecting duct. (This same type of effect of alkalosis on potassium concentration in nonrenal cells was described earlier in this chapter.) The presence of an alkalosis somehow stimulates the basolateral potassium-entry step.

What about the presence of an acidosis—does it do just the opposite, i.e., reduce potassium secretion and thereby cause potassium retention?

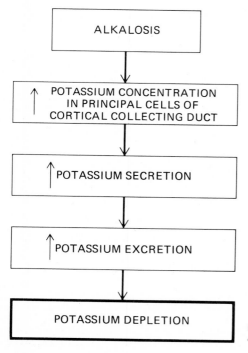

Figure 8-7 Pathway by which alkalosis causes potassium depletion.

For respiratory acidosis and certain forms of metabolic acidosis, the answer is yes, but only during the most acute states, usually less than 24 h. In other forms of metabolic acidosis there may not even be an acute retention phase. But the really surprising fact is that even respiratory acidosis and those forms of metabolic acidosis that do manifest acute reductions in potassium excretion usually come ultimately to manifest *increased* potassium secretion. Attempts have been made to explain these phenomena,[10] but at the moment the mechanisms by which chronic acidosis alters renal potassium handling remain unclear.

Finally, it should be emphasized that the relationships described here are only one side of the coin. We shall describe in the next chapter how primary changes in potassium balance induce secondary changes in the renal handling of hydrogen ions.

Study questions: 60 to 63

[10] See Gennari and Cohen in Suggested Readings.

9

RENAL REGULATION OF HYDROGEN-ION BALANCE

OBJECTIVES

The student describes the sources of hydrogen-ion gain and loss, states the major bodily buffer systems, writes the Henderson-Hasselbalch equation for the CO_2-bicarbonate buffer system, and states in general terms the role of the kidneys in regulating extracellular pH.

The student understands the renal excretion of bicarbonate.
1   States the three renal processes that determine bicarbonate excretion
2   Calculates the mass of bicarbonate filtered each day
3   Describes the acidifying effect of renal bicarbonate loss
4   Describes the mechanism by which tubular bicarbonate reabsorption occurs; states the role of carbonic anhydrase; quantifies the contributions of the proximal and distal nephron segments to bicarbonate reabsorption
5   Describes the mechanism of bicarbonate secretion and the situation in which it occurs

The student understands how the kidneys add new bicarbonate to the blood, i.e., excrete hydrogen ions.
1   Describes how tubular hydrogen-ion secretion can add new bicarbonate to the blood, i.e., lead to the excretion of hydrogen ion
2   States the limiting urine pH and its significance
3   States the major luminal nonbicarbonate buffer and its normal rate of excretion
4   States what determines whether a secreted hydrogen ion combines in the lumen with a filtered bicarbonate or a nonbicarbonate buffer
5   Describes how proximal-tubular production of NH_4^+ from glutamine, followed by excretion of the NH_4^+ in the urine, contributes to the addition of new bicarbonate to the blood
6   Defines titratable acid
7   Calculates, given data, the rate at which the kidneys contribute new bicarbonate to the blood

The student understands the homeostatic control of renal acid-base compensation.
1   States the control of renal glutamine metabolism and NH_4^+ excretion
2   States the control of tubular hydrogen-ion secretion by P_{CO_2}, local extracellular pH, and aldosterone; states the effect of metabolic acidosis on aldosterone secretion
3   Lists the changes (increase or decrease) of acid secretion, titratable acid excretion, bicarbonate excretion, NH_4^+ excretion, renal addition of new bicarbonate to the blood, and plasma bicarbonate in metabolic acidosis, metabolic alkalosis, respiratory acidosis, and respiratory alkalosis

The student understands how various factors can cause the kidneys to generate or maintain a metabolic alkalosis.
1   Describes the influence of extracellular volume contraction and chloride depletion on bicarbonate reabsorption and the capacity of the kidneys to repair an alkalosis
2   States the effect of increased aldosterone alone on hydrogen-ion secretion
3   States the effect of severe potassium depletion alone on hydrogen-ion secretion
4   Describes how a combination of aldosterone excess and potassium depletion generates a metabolic alkalosis

The regulation of total-body hydrogen-ion balance can be viewed in the same way as the balance of any other ion—as the matching of gains and losses (Table 9-1). Not shown in the table is the gastrointestinal absorption of ingested acids or bases, which is usually a negligible factor (except in individuals who deliberately ingest large quantities of bicarbonate or some other acid or base).

Normally, the major route for gain is the metabolic generation of hydrogen ions within the body. A huge quantity of CO_2 (15,000 to 20,000 mmols) is generated daily as the result of oxidative metabolism and yields hydrogen ions via these reactions:

$$CO_2 + H_2O \longrightarrow H_2CO_3 \longrightarrow HCO_3^- + H^+ \qquad (9\text{-}1)$$

But this source does not normally constitute a net gain of hydrogen ions since all those hydrogen ions generated via these reactions during passage of blood through the tissues are reincorporated into water when the reactions are reversed during passage of blood through the lungs. Net retention of CO_2, however, as in hypoventilation, does result in a net gain of hydrogen ions. Conversely, net loss of CO_2, as in hyperventilation, causes net elimination of hydrogen ions.

The body also produces acids, both organic and inorganic, from sources other than CO_2. These are termed **nonvolatile acids** or **fixed acids**, to distinguish them from those produced from CO_2. These acids include phosphoric acid and sulfuric acid generated during the catabolism of proteins and other organic molecules containing sulfur and phosphorus,

Table 9-1 Sources of Hydrogen-Ion Gain and Loss

GAIN

1. Generation of hydrogen ions from CO_2
2. Production of acids from the metabolism of protein and other organic molecules
3. Gain of hydrogen ions because of loss of bicarbonate in diarrhea or other nongastric gastrointestinal fluids
4. Gain of hydrogen ions because of loss of bicarbonate in the urine

LOSS

1. Loss of hydrogen ions in vomitus
2. Loss of hydrogen ions in urine

as well as lactic acid, ketone bodies, and others. In the United States, where the diet is high in protein, people normally have a net daily production of 40 to 80 mmols of nonvolatile acids. In contrast, in people whose diet is mainly vegetarian, there is a net metabolic production of bicarbonate rather than hydrogen ions; i.e., the nonvolatile metabolic contribution is actually one of net loss of hydrogen ions.[1]

A third potential source of net bodily gain or loss of hydrogen ion is the gastrointestinal secretions leaving the body. Vomitus contains a high concentration of hydrogen ions and so constitutes a source of net loss. In contrast, the other gastrointestinal secretions are alkaline, i.e., contain a higher concentration of bicarbonate than exists in plasma. Loss of these fluids, as in diarrhea, constitutes, in essence, a bodily gain of hydrogen ions. This is a very important point: Given the reversible equations shown in Eq. 9-1, the *loss* of a bicarbonate ion from the body has virtually the same net result as *gaining* a hydrogen ion because loss of the bicarbonate causes the reactions to be driven to the right, thereby generating a hydrogen ion. Similarly, the *gain* of bicarbonate by the body has virtually the same net result as *losing* a hydrogen ion because the reaction will be driven to the left.

Finally, the urine constitutes the fourth source of net hydrogen-ion gain or loss. As is the case for the other inorganic ions described in this book, the renal excretion of hydrogen ions is regulated to achieve a stable balance and, hence, maintain a relatively stable hydrogen-ion concentra-

---

[1] Another large potential source of bicarbonate is protein catabolism to NH_4^+ and HCO_3^-. The NH_4^+ will not dissociate, to any significant degree, to yield hydrogen ions because the pK of the $NH_4^+ \rightleftharpoons NH_3 + H^+$ reaction is very high (9.2); accordingly protein catabolism yields net HCO_3^-. However, virtually all the NH_4^+ and HCO_3^- formed by protein catabolism are rapidly combined to form urea in the liver, and so the HCO_3^- disappears. In other words, urea formation undoes the alkalinizing effects of protein catabolism. (We will revisit this issue, this time in the text, in the section on ammonium.) This glib explanation of how protein catabolism doesn't yield net bicarbonate, however, is not accepted by all. Indeed, some have argued that the control of ureagenesis is the major regulator of acid-base balance. These scientists go so far as to argue that the kidneys play little if any role in acid-base balance (if they are right, you could simply skip the rest of this chapter). For details on this fascinating controversy, see articles by Atkinson, Knepper et al., and Walser, in Suggested Readings.

tion of the extracellular fluid. Thus, the kidneys normally excrete the 40 to 80 mmols of hydrogen ion generated by the average American diet. In contrast, they excrete the required amount of bicarbonate in a person whose metabolism is generating net alkali rather than net hydrogen ion. The kidneys also adjust their excretion of hydrogen ion and bicarbonate to compensate for any net retention or elimination of CO_2, for any increase in the metabolic production of hydrogen ions (as in diabetic ketoacidosis, for example), and for any increased loss of hydrogen ion or bicarbonate via the gastrointestinal tract.

The idea that hydrogen-ion regulation involves the same kind of input-output balancing as does that of sodium and other ions is easily obscured by the phenomenon of buffering. Between their generation and their elimination, most hydrogen ions are buffered by extracellular and intracellular buffers; i.e., they seem to disappear in a way that sodium ions do not. The normal extracellular fluid pH of 7.4 corresponds to an actual hydrogen-ion concentration of only 40 nanomol/L. Without buffering interposed between generation and excretion, the daily turnover rate of only the nonvolatile acids—amounting to many millimols (1 millimol = 1 million nanomols)—would cause large changes in pH. Buffering minimizes changes in hydrogen-ion concentration but does not actually eliminate the hydrogen ions from the body or retain them. This is the function of the kidneys.

The only important *extracellular* buffer is the CO_2-HCO_3^- system. The major *intracellular* buffers are phosphates and proteins, including hemoglobin. Because all these buffer systems are in equilibrium with one another, a change in one buffer pair will be associated with changes in the others. Accordingly, even though the intracellular buffers account for 50 to 90 percent of the buffering of excess hydrogen ions (depending on the source of the hydrogen ions), the emphasis in describing the overall regulation of the pH of the bodily fluids is, for a variety of reasons, generally on the CO_2-HCO_3^- system.

The major reason for doing so is that there are extremely precise physiological mechanisms for regulating the two critical components of the CO_2-HCO_3^- system; the P_{CO_2} is regulated by the respiratory system, and the plasma bicarbonate concentration by the kidneys. As should be evident from the Henderson-Hasselbalch form of the equation, regulation of the P_{CO_2} and bicarbonate concentration achieves regulation of the pH:

$$pH = 6.1 + \log HCO_3^- /0.03\ P_{CO_2}$$

To reiterate, the kidneys contribute to the homeostasis of extracellular fluid hydrogen-ion concentration by regulating plasma bicarbonate concentration. They do so in two ways: (1) excretion of filtered and/or secreted bicarbonate and (2) addition of *new* bicarbonate to the plasma flowing through the kidneys. Either the kidneys can lower plasma bicarbonate concentration by excreting bicarbonate in the urine or they can raise plasma bicarbonate concentration by "producing" new bicarbonate and adding it to the blood flowing through the kidneys.

Thus, in response to a lowering of plasma hydrogen-ion concentration (**alkalosis**), the kidneys excrete large quantities of bicarbonate in the urine, thereby raising plasma hydrogen-ion concentration (recall that the excretion of a bicarbonate in the urine has virtually the same effect on the blood as would adding a hydrogen ion to the blood).

In contrast, in response to a rise in plasma hydrogen-ion concentration (**acidosis**), the kidneys do not excrete bicarbonate in the urine but instead add new bicarbonate to the blood, thereby lowering the plasma hydrogen-ion concentration. As we shall see, the renal addition of new bicarbonate to the blood is associated with the excretion of an equal amount of hydrogen ions in the urine. "The kidney has added new bicarbonate to the blood" and "The kidney has *excreted* acid" are synonymous statements. Thus, to compensate for acidosis, the kidneys excrete acid urine and alkalinize the blood; in response to alkalosis, they excrete bicarbonate-containing alkaline urine and acidify the blood.

Let us now look at how the kidneys perform these actions—either bicarbonate excretion or bicarbonate addition to the blood.

BICARBONATE EXCRETION

Urinary bicarbonate excretion is the result of bicarbonate filtration, reabsorption, and secretion:

$$\text{Excreted } HCO_3^-/\text{day} = HCO_3^- \text{ filtered} + HCO_3^- \text{ secreted} - HCO_3^- \text{ reabsorbed}$$

For the moment we shall ignore bicarbonate secretion and focus only on filtration and reabsorption.

Bicarbonate Filtration and Reabsorption

Bicarbonate is completely filterable at the glomerulus. How much is normally filtered per day?

$$\begin{aligned} \text{Filtered } HCO_3^-/\text{day} &= GFR \times P_{HCO_3^-} \\ &= 180 \text{ L/day} \times 24 \text{ mmoles/L} \\ &= 4320 \text{ mmoles/day} \end{aligned}$$

Excretion of this bicarbonate would be tantamount to adding more than 4 L of 1 N acid to the body. In individuals on an average American diet, virtually all is reabsorbed. Thus, the reabsorption of bicarbonate is normally a conservation process, and little if any appears in the urine.

Bicarbonate reabsorption is an active process, but it is not accomplished in the conventional manner of simply having an active pump for bicarbonate ions at either the luminal or basolateral membrane. Rather, the mechanism by which bicarbonate is reabsorbed involves the tubular secretion of hydrogen ions. Let us look first at the basic process of hydrogen-ion secretion and then apply it to bicarbonate reabsorption.

Hydrogen secretion occurs in the proximal tubule and collecting-duct system.[2] Recall that the collecting ducts contain both intercalated and principal cells; the latter reabsorb sodium and secrete potassium, whereas the intercalated cells secrete hydrogen ion (they also can reabsorb potassium). As shown in Fig. 9-1A, within proximal cells and intercalated cells a hydrogen ion and a hydroxyl ion are generated from water. The hydrogen ion is actively secreted into the tubular lumen; this is achieved in the proximal cells by a Na,H countertransporter (Fig. 6-1) and in the intercalated cells by a primary H-ATPase pump. The hydroxyl ion left behind inside the cell combines with CO_2 to form a bicarbonate ion, in a reaction catalyzed by **carbonic anhydrase**. The bicarbonate moves downhill across the basolateral membrane into the interstitial fluid and, then, into the blood.[3] The net result is that for every hydrogen ion secreted into the lumen, a bicarbonate ion enters the blood in the peritubular capillaries.

Although the pathway illustrated in Fig. 9-1A is biochemically the most likely one followed, we shall use in subsequent figures the more traditional pathway shown in Fig. 9-1B. In this schema, the hydrogen ion to be secreted is generated from H_2CO_3, and the role of carbonic anhydrase is to catalyze the formation of H_2CO_3 from H_2O and CO_2. We have chosen to use this schema because it is easier to visualize, and it retains a role for carbonic anhydrase more familiar to the student.

Figure 9-2 illustrates how the overall process of hydrogen-ion secretion achieves bicarbonate reabsorption. Note that the intracellular events are identical to those shown in Fig. 9-1—a hydrogen ion is secreted into the lumen while the bicarbonate generated in the cell moves across the basolateral membrane and into the blood. Once in the tubular lumen, the secreted hydrogen ion combines with a *filtered bicarbonate* to form carbonic acid. This breaks down to water and carbon dioxide, which diffuse into the cell (and can be used by the cell in another cycle). The overall result is that the bicarbonate filtered from the blood at the renal corpuscle has disappeared, but its place in the blood has been taken by the bicarbonate that was produced inside the cell, and so no net change in

---

[2] The ascending thick loop of Henle may also secrete some hydrogen ion (see Madsen and Tisher in Suggested Readings).

[3] The bicarbonate exit step across the basolateral membrane differs in the proximal tubule and collecting-duct system. In the former, it is mainly via Na^+/HCO_3^- cotransport, whereas in the latter, it is mainly via Cl^-/HCO_3^- countertransport (see articles by Gluck, Levine and Jacobson, and Steinmetz in Suggested Readings).

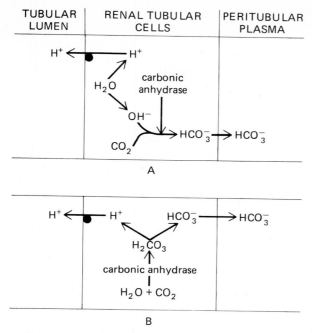

Figure 9-1   Two views of hydrogen-ion secretion by proximal tubular cells and intercalated cells in the collecting duct system. In both (1) a hydrogen ion is formed in the cell and secreted into the lumen; (2) a bicarbonate ion enters the peritubular plasma from the cell; (3) carbonic anhydrase catalyzes the essential reaction. For simplicity, the mechanism for the active transport of the hydrogen ion across the luminal membrane and the downhill movement of bicarbonate across the basolateral membrane are not shown in the figure. In the proximal tubule, hydrogen-ion secretion is via a Na, H countertransporter (Fig. 6-1), whereas in the intercalated cells it is via a primary H-ATPase pump.

plasma bicarbonate concentration has occurred. It may seem inaccurate to refer to this process as bicarbonate "reabsorption" since the bicarbonate that appears in the peritubular plasma is not the same bicarbonate ion that was filtered. Yet the overall result is, in effect, the same as it would be if the filtered bicarbonate had been more conventionally reabsorbed, like a sodium or potassium ion.

It is also important to note that the hydrogen ion that was *secreted* into the lumen is *not excreted* in the urine. It has been incorporated into water. The key point here is that any secreted hydrogen ion that combines with bicarbonate in the lumen to effect bicarbonate reabsorption does not contribute to the urinary excretion of acid.

As noted earlier, the process of hydrogen-ion secretion and bicarbonate reabsorption occurs in both the proximal tubule and collecting-duct system. Quantitatively, the proximal tubule is most important in that it reabsorbs approximately 80 to 90 percent of the filtered bicarbonate. The remaining bicarbonate is normally reabsorbed by the collecting-duct system. Throughout the tubule, as shown in Fig. 9-1, *intracellular* carbonic

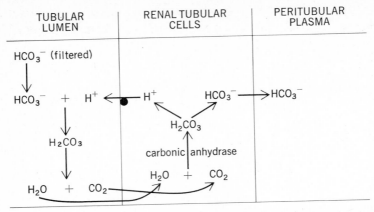

Figure 9-2 General mechanism by which filtered bicarbonate is reabsorbed by proximal tubular cells and by intercalated cells in the collecting duct system. In studying this figure, begin with the carbon dioxide and water in the tubular cells. As noted in Fig. 9-1, hydrogen-ion movement across the luminal membrane is via a Na, H countertransporter in the proximal tubule (Fig. 6-1), whereas in the intercalated cells it is via a primary H-ATPase pump. Also not shown in the figure is the fact that in the proximal tubule but not in the cortical collecting duct, the breakdown of H_2CO_3 to CO_2 and H_2O *in the lumen* is catalyzed by carbonic anhydrase present in the luminal membrane.

anhydrase is involved in the reactions generating hydrogen ion and bicarbonate. In the proximal tubule, carbonic anhydrase is *also* located in the luminal cell membranes, and this carbonic anhydrase catalyzes the *intraluminal* decomposition of the very large quantities of carbonic acid formed in this tubular segment. The collecting-duct system does not have luminal-membrane carbonic anhydrase.[4]

Bicarbonate Secretion

As described above, the intercalated cells of the cortical collecting duct reabsorb bicarbonate, but under certain circumstances this nephron segment may manifest net secretion, rather than net reabsorption, because a particular population of intercalated cells can secrete bicarbonate.[5] The

[4] Because of this absence, the intraluminal breakdown of H_2CO_3 to CO_2 and H_2O occurs relatively slowly in these segments. Therefore, much of the CO_2 formation occurs after the urine has left the tubule and entered the lower urinary tract. Here, the surface-to-volume relationships are unfavorable for the diffusion of CO_2 out of the lumen. Accordingly, for this reason (and others not mentioned here), the urine P_{CO_2} can be much higher than the arterial P_{CO_2} under certain conditions. (See Dubose, Jr., and Gennari et al., in Suggested Readings.)

[5] It is not clear whether this population is entirely distinct from the intercalated cells that secrete hydrogen ions or whether a single population of intercalated cells can be transformed back and forth from hydrogen-ion secretors to bicarbonate secretors. See articles by Madsen and Tisher and by Steinmetz in Suggested Readings.

mechanism of secretion can be visualized by taking the same intracellular events shown in Fig. 9-1A but exchanging the membranes that the transport processes are on. Thus, in a bicarbonate-secreting intercalated cell, the H-ATPase pump is located on the basolateral membrane, whereas the bicarbonate transporter (a Cl^-/HCO_3^- countertransporter) is on the luminal membrane (see Appendix B). Accordingly, bicarbonate enters the tubular lumen while hydrogen ion enters the blood, where it can combine with a bicarbonate ion in the plasma. Thus, the overall process achieves disappearance of plasma bicarbonate and excretion of bicarbonate in the urine, with resulting acidification of the plasma.

The one situation in which the cortical collecting duct manifests net secretion of bicarbonate rather than net reabsorption is alkalosis. However, even during alkalosis, the net handling of bicarbonate for the *entire* tubule is always reabsorption, never secretion. In other words, any bicarbonate secreted by the cortical collecting ducts during alkalosis is considerably less than the amount of bicarbonate being reabsorbed by the proximal tubule and medullary collecting duct.

Because bicarbonate reabsorption is always the predominant process for the *entire* tubule, in the rest of this chapter we shall refer, for the sake of simplicity, only to *reabsorption,* using this term to denote "net reabsorption"—the result of bicarbonate reabsorption and secretion. We shall not try (the experimental data are usually not available) to quantify the contribution of the two unidirectional movements to the changes in net reabsorption.

This completes our survey of bicarbonate excretion. Now we turn to the second way in which the kidneys can regulate plasma bicarbonate, namely, the contribution of new bicarbonate to the blood.

ADDITION OF NEW BICARBONATE TO THE PLASMA (RENAL EXCRETION OF ACID)

Besides being able to conserve all the filtered bicarbonate, the kidneys can also contribute *new* bicarbonate to the plasma, so that the mass of bicarbonate leaving the kidneys via the renal veins exceeds that entering the kidneys via the arteries. The effect of adding new bicarbonate to the body is, of course, to alkalinize it, and this is the renal compensation for acidosis.

There are two mechanisms by which the kidneys add new bicarbonate to the body: (1) secretion of hydrogen ions, which instead of effecting bicarbonate reabsorption, are excreted in the urine, combined with non-bicarbonate buffers supplied by filtration; (2) catabolism of glutamine in association with excretion of ammonium in the urine. We shall now describe these two mechanisms.

Hydrogen-Ion Secretion and Excretion on Urinary Buffers

We have seen how hydrogen-ion secretion achieves bicarbonate reab-sorption and how this process prevents loss of filtered bicarbonate but adds no new bicarbonate to the blood. Now we shall see that the identical process of hydrogen-ion secretion can also achieve hydrogen-ion excre-tion and addition of new bicarbonate to the blood. Which result—either bicarbonate reabsorption or contribution of new bicarbonate to the blood—is achieved by the secreted hydrogen ion is determined solely by the fate of this ion within the tubular lumen.

In the case of bicarbonate reabsorption, as we have seen, the se-creted hydrogen ion combines with filtered bicarbonate and is incorpo-rated into water. In contrast, in the case of new bicarbonate addition to the blood, the secreted hydrogen ion combines with nonbicarbonate buff-ers in the lumen (or to an extremely small degree, remains free in solution) and is excreted. Normally, the most important of these buffers is phos-phate, more specifically HPO_4^{2-}.

Figure 9-3 illustrates the sequence of events that achieves hydrogen-ion excretion on phosphate and the addition of new bicarbonate to the blood. The process of hydrogen-ion secretion in this sequence is exactly the same as that described previously (Fig. 9-1), but the net overall effect is different simply because the secreted hydrogen ion reacts in the lumen with filtered phosphate rather than with filtered bicarbonate. Therefore, the bicarbonate generated within the tubular cell and entering the plasma constitutes a *net gain* of bicarbonate by the blood, not merely a replace-ment for a filtered bicarbonate. Thus, when a secreted hydrogen ion combines in the lumen with a buffer other than bicarbonate, the overall effect is not merely one of bicarbonate conservation but rather of addition to the blood of a new bicarbonate, which raises the bicarbonate con-centration of the blood and alkalinizes it.

The figure also demonstrates another important point; namely, that the renal contribution of new bicarbonate to the blood is accompanied by the *excretion* of an equivalent amount of hydrogen ion, buffered by phosphate, in the urine. In this case, in contrast to the reabsorption of bicarbonate, the *secreted* hydrogen ion remains in the tubular fluid, trapped there by the phosphate buffer, and is *excreted* in the urine. This should reinforce the concept that when the kidneys add new bicarbonate to the blood, they are really excreting hydrogen ion from the body, thereby alkalinizing it. It must be emphasized at this point that glomerular filtration of hydrogen ions makes no signifcant contribution to hydrogen-ion excretion because the concentration of free hydrogen ion at a pH of 7.4, the pH of glomerular filtrate, is less than $10^{-7}M$. Even multiplying this figure by 180L/day, one comes up with less than 0.1 mmol filtered per day.

The type and quantity of nonbicarbonate buffers are important deter-minants of the maximal rate at which the kidneys can excrete acid (con-

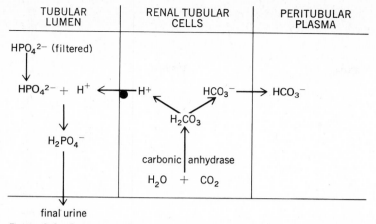

Figure 9-3 Reaction of secreted hydrogen ion with filtered phosphate. Note that a new bicarbonate ion has been released into the blood. In contrast, Fig. 9-2 shows that no net gain or loss of blood bicarbonate occurs when the secreted hydrogen ion is used for bicarbonate reabsorption.

tribute new bicarbonate to the blood). This stems from the fact that for reasons that need not concern us here, net addition of hydrogen ions to the lumen ceases when a maximal luminal hydrogen-ion concentration—a pH of approximately 4.4—is reached.[6] The urinary buffers react with secreted hydrogen ions and prevent this limiting concentration for free hydrogen ion from being reached.

Phosphate and Organic Acids as Buffers To repeat, phosphate is normally the most important nonbicarbonate urinary buffer. The relationship between monobasic and dibasic phosphate is as follows:

$$HPO_4^{2-} + H^+ \rightleftharpoons H_2PO_4^-$$

This buffer pair provides an excellent buffer system for urine because its pK is 6.8. Expressed in Henderson-Hasselbalch terms,

$$pH = 6.8 + \log HPO_4^{2-}/H_2PO_4^-$$

At the normal pH of plasma and, therefore, of the glomerular filtrate, the equation becomes

$$7.4 = 6.8 + \log HPO_4^{2-}/H_2PO_4^-$$

Solving the equation, we find that there is four times more dibasic (HPO_4^{2-}) than monobasic ($H_2PO_4^-$) phosphate in plasma, and this HPO_4^{2-}

[6] See Steinmetz in Suggested Readings.

is available for buffering secreted hydrogen ions. By the time the minimal intratubular pH of 4.4 is reached, virtually all the HPO_4^{2-} has been converted to $H_2PO_4^-$.

How much HPO_4^{2-} is normally filtered per day?[7]

$$\text{Filtered total phosphate/day} = 180 \text{ L/day} \times 1 \text{ mmol/L}$$
$$= 180 \text{ mmol/day}$$
$$\text{Filtered } HPO_4^{2-} = 80\% \times 180 \text{ mmol/day}$$
$$= 144 \text{ mmol/day}$$

Not all this filtered HPO_4^{2-} is available for buffering, however, because about 75 percent of filtered phosphate is reabsorbed. Accordingly, unreabsorbed HPO_4^{2-} available for buffering is 0.25×144 mmol/day $= 36$ mmol/day. Thus, the reabsorption of phosphate considerably limits the supply of HPO_4^{2-} for buffering. It is adaptive, therefore, that the presence of a low plasma pH (acidosis) partially inhibits phosphate reabsorption,[8] thereby increasing the amount of luminal phosphate available for buffering. This effect is relatively modest, however, and so during severe acidosis, the second mechanism for renal production of new bicarbonate—glutamine metabolism—usually bears most of the compensatory burden.

Under certain conditions, various organic buffers may appear in the tubular fluid in large enough quantities to allow them also to act as important buffers. A particularly interesting example is the patient with uncontrolled diabetes mellitus. As a result of insulin deficiency, such a patient may become extremely acidotic because he or she produces large quantities of acetoacetic acid and β-hydroxybutyric acid, which at plasma pH almost completely dissociate to yield anions (β-hydroxybutyrate and acetoacetate) and hydrogen ions. These anions are filtered at the renal corpuscle but are only partly reabsorbed because they are present in great enough quantities to exceed the renal reabsorptive T_ms for them. Accordingly, they are available in the tubular fluid to buffer a portion of the hydrogen ions being secreted by the tubules to compensate for the acidosis. However, their usefulness in this role is limited by the fact that their pKs are low—approximately 4.5. This means that only about half of these anions will be titrated by secreted hydrogen ions before the limiting urine pH of 4.4 is reached; i.e., only half of them can actually be used as buffers.

---

[7] The number, 1 mM in the equation that follows, is the value of phosphate in glomerular filtrate; it is somewhat lower than the plasma concentration because a small fraction of plasma phosphate is protein-bound and, therefore, not filterable.

[8] See Hamm and Simon in Suggested Readings for mechanisms.

Qualitative Integration of Bicarbonate Reabsorption and Hydrogen-Ion Excretion on Nonbicarbonate Buffers To repeat, a hydrogen ion secreted by the tubule can suffer one of two general fates: (1) It can combine with filtered bicarbonate, in which case the overall process accomplishes bicarbonate reabsorption, or (2) it can combine with filtered nonbicarbonate buffers such as phosphate. The first case is a conservation process, by which the kidneys prevent loss of bicarbonate from the body. This process alone does not alkalinize the body but rather prevents the development of an acidosis caused by bicarbonate loss. In contrast, the second process contributes new bicarbonate to the body and simultaneously excretes acid, thereby alkalinizing the body.

What determines whether the secreted hydrogen ions, once in the lumen, combine with bicarbonate, on the one hand, or with phosphate and organic buffers, on the other? This depends on the pKs of each buffer-pair reaction and on the concentrations of each buffer present. To simplify matters, one may assume that compared to bicarbonate, relatively little nonbicarbonate buffer is titrated, i.e., combines with hydrogen ion, until most of the bicarbonate has been reabsorbed. This is true mainly because the concentration of bicarbonate in the glomerular filtrate is so much higher than the concentrations of the other buffers. Once most of the filtered bicarbonate has been reabsorbed, the secreted hydrogen ions combine with the other buffers.

This analysis also explains the contributions of the different nephron segments to these processes. The proximal tubule secretes many more hydrogen ions than does the collecting-duct system, and most of these proximally secreted hydrogen ions go to achieve bicarbonate reabsorption; as stated in Chap. 6, 90 percent of filtered bicarbonate is reabsorbed proximally. Because most of the secreted hydrogen ions are used for bicarbonate reabsorption, the pH of the luminal fluid falls less than 1 pH unit, and only a small amount of hydrogen ion is picked up by phosphate and organic buffers. In contrast, because relatively little of the filtered bicarbonate normally remains by the beginning of the collecting-duct system, the hydrogen ions secreted by the collecting-duct system can reabsorb this bicarbonate and then create the lower pH required for titration of nonbicarbonate urinary buffers. However, should a large amount of bicarbonate escape proximal reabsorption, most of the hydrogen ions secreted by the collecting-duct system, too, would be expended in reabsorbing bicarbonate rather than in titrating urinary buffers.

Glutamine Catabolism and NH_4^+ Excretion

The cells of the proximal tubule (and to a much lesser extent, other nephron segments) extract glutamine from both the glomerular filtrate and peritubular blood and hydrolyse it to glutamate ion and NH_4^+. Most of the

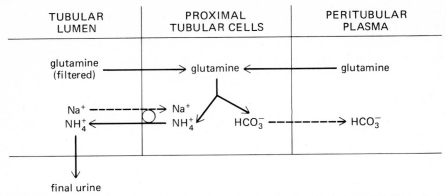

Figure 9-4 Ammonium production and secretion by proximal tubular cells. Glutamine moves into the cells across both the luminal and basolateral membranes and is metabolized, yielding ammonium and bicarbonate. The ammonium is actively secreted into the lumen via a Na, NH_4^+ countertransporter, and the bicarbonate moves across the basolateral membrane and into the peritubular plasma.

glutamate is metabolized to alpha-ketoglutarate, with the liberation of another NH_4^+. The subsequent metabolism of the alpha-ketoglutarate, either to glucose or to CO_2 and water, yields two bicarbonates. Thus, the overall yield of NH_4^+ and bicarbonate from glutamine can be written,

$$1 \text{ glutamine} \rightarrow 2 \text{ } NH_4^+ + 2 \text{ } HCO_3^-$$

The NH_4^+ is actively secreted into the lumen and excreted, whereas the bicarbonate moves into the peritubular capillaries and constitutes *new* bicarbonate (Fig. 9-4).[9]

It is absolutely essential for the NH_4^+ produced from glutamine to be excreted, rather than to enter the blood, for the bicarbonate released into the blood truly to constitute a net gain of bicarbonate to the body. First, let us point out an intuitively seductive but *wrong* possible explanation for this statement. You might think that if NH_4^+ were to enter the blood along with the bicarbonate, the NH_4^+ would directly donate a proton to the bicarbonate to yield NH_3, CO_2, and H_2O, but this cannot happen to any significant degree. Why? Because the pK of the $NH_4^+ \rightleftharpoons NH_3 + H^+$ reaction is so high (9.2), NH_4^+ donates virtually no protons at physiological pHs; i.e., NH_4^+ is not really an acid at these pHs.

What, then, is the correct explanation for the fact that the NH_4^+ must be excreted for the bicarbonate to remain in the blood? The reason is that were both the NH_4^+ and the bicarbonate to enter the blood, they would

---

[9] The active secretion of NH_4^+ is achieved by a Na,NH_4^+ countertransporter, whereas the movement of HCO_3^- across the basolateral membrane is via a 3 HCO_3^-,Na cotransporter. (See Knepper et al. in Suggested Readings.)

rapidly be reincorporated into urea or glutamine in the liver, with the disappearance of the bicarbonate.[10]

A comparison of Figs. 9-3 and 9-4 demonstrates that the overall result—renal contribution of a new bicarbonate to the blood—is the same regardless of whether it is achieved by H^+ secretion and excretion on buffers (Fig. 9-3) or by glutamine metabolism with NH_4^+ excretion (Fig. 9-4). It is convenient, therefore, to view the latter case as representing H^+ "bound" to NH_3, just as the former case constitutes H^+ bound to phosphate or other nonbicarbonate buffers. In this manner, we can in both cases quantitatively equate the terms "H^+ excretion" and "renal contribution of new bicarbonate."

To reiterate, the NH_4^+ formed by the proximal tubular cells must be excreted if the bicarbonate simultaneously formed and moved into the blood is to remain new bicarbonate. In fact, most of the NH_4^+ produced is, indeed, secreted into the lumen (a small fraction enters the blood, instead, and so is "wasted"), and almost all this NH_4^+ is ultimately excreted. The story would be simple if this proximally secreted NH_4^+ merely flowed the length of the tubule to be excreted. In reality, however, the tubular handling of NH_4^+ beyond the proximal tubule actually is a very complex sequence of transport events.[11] The only important point for us is that almost all the NH_4^+ formed by the proximal tubule does end up being excreted.

QUANTITATION OF RENAL ACID-BASE COMPENSATION

Now we can quantitate the kidneys' contribution to hydrogen-ion balance. Said in another way, we can calculate the kidneys' net bicarbonate addition to or elimination from the body. This value is, to say it again, identical to the kidneys' net excretion of acid.

Such a calculation is made by answering three questions:

1 How much bicarbonate is excreted in the urine? This represents bicarbonate *loss* from the body. It is measured simply by multiplying the urinary flow rate by the urinary bicarbonate concentration.

2 How much *new* bicarbonate is contributed to the plasma by secretion of hydrogen ions that end up combining in the tubular lumen

---

[10] To emphasize these points, let us explain why the administration of NH_4Cl causes acidosis. As described in the text, the NH_4^+ that appears when the NH_4Cl dissociates does not yield H^+ and NH_3 to any significant degree. Rather, the NH_4^+ is incorporated into urea and/or glutamine, and these reactions utilize bicarbonate from the plasma. It is this disappearance of bicarbonate that causes the acidosis.

[11] These events, involving movement of both NH_3 and NH_4^+, include transport from the ascending loop into the interstitium, countercurrent multiplication in the medulla, and finally, secretion into the collecting ducts. See Hamm and Simon, and Knepper et al., in Suggested Readings.

with nonbicarbonate urinary buffers? This can be measured by titrating the urine with NaOH to a pH of 7.4, the pH of the plasma from which the glomerular filtrate originated. This simply reverses the events that occurred within the tubular lumen when the tubular fluid was titrated by secreted hydrogen ions. Thus, the number of milliequivalents of sodium hydroxide required to reach pH 7.4 must equal the number of milliequivalents of hydrogen ion added to the tubular fluid that combined with phosphate and organic buffers. This value is known as the **titratable acid.** It must be stressed that the titratable-acid measurement does *not* pick up hydrogen ions in NH_4^+. The reason is that the pK of the ammonia-ammonium reaction is so high (9.2) that titration with alkali to pH 7.4 will not remove hydrogen ions from NH_4^+.

   3 How much *new* bicarbonate is contributed by glutamine metabolism with NH_4^+ excretion? This can be calculated by measuring urinary NH_4^+ excretion (urine flow rate × urinary NH_4^+ concentration) since for every NH_4^+ excreted, a new bicarbonate was contributed to the blood.

   Thus, the data required for a quantitative assessment of the renal contribution to acid-base regulation in any person are

   1 Titratable acid excreted
   2 *plus* NH_4^+ excreted
   3 *minus* HCO_3^- excreted (i.e., filtered HCO_3^- lost from the body because of incomplete reabsorption plus HCO_3^- secretion)

   Total = net HCO_3^- gain or loss to the body (negative values equal loss, positive values equal gain)

Note that there is no term for free hydrogen ion in the urine because, even at a minimal urine pH of 4.4, the number of free hydrogen ions is trivial.

   Typical urine data for the amounts of bicarbonate contributed to the blood by the kidneys in the three potential acid-base states are as follows:

Alkalosis

Titratable acid = 0 mmoles/day
Plus excreted NH_4^+ = 0 mmoles/day
Minus excreted HCO_3^- = 80 mmoles/day
Total = −80 mmoles/day (80 mmoles bicarbonate *lost* from body) (urine pH = 8.0)

Normal state

Titratable acid = 20 mmoles/day
Plus excreted NH_4^+ = 40 mmoles/day
Minus excreted HCO_3^- = 1 mmole/day
Total = 59 mmoles/day (59 mmoles bicarbonate *added* to body) (urine pH = 6.0)

Acidosis

$$\begin{aligned}
\text{Titratable acid} &= 40 \text{ mmoles/day} \\
\text{Plus excreted } NH_4^+ &= 160 \text{ mmoles/day} \\
\text{Minus excreted } HCO_3^- &= 0 \text{ mmoles/day} \\
\text{Total} &= 200 \text{ mmoles/day (200 mmoles bicarbonate} \\
&\quad \textit{added} \text{ to body) (urine pH } = 4.6)
\end{aligned}$$

It should be emphasized that the data shown for alkalosis are typical of respiratory alkalosis and "pure" metabolic alkalosis, i.e., alkalosis uncomplicated by other electrolyte abnormalities. As we shall see in subsequent sections, electrolyte imbalances frequently complicate the picture in metabolic alkalosis, so that the expected values are not seen.

HOMEOSTATIC CONTROL OF RENAL ACID-BASE COMPENSATION

The patterns given in the previous section are what one would predict for renal compensation for altered hydrogen-ion balance, and now we must describe the control mechanisms that account for these patterns. What actually causes bicarbonate excretion to be increased in alkalosis and zero in acidosis? What causes the excretion of titratable acid and NH_4^+ to show just the opposite pattern?

Multiple factors control the various renal processes that determine net renal contribution to plasma bicarbonate (Table 9-2). We mentioned two earlier: (1) the inhibition of phosphate reabsorption that occurs during acidosis and (2) the occurrence of bicarbonate secretion by the cortical collecting duct during alkalosis. However, the major physiological controls operate on glutamine metabolism and NH_4^+ excretion and on tubular hydrogen-ion secretion.

Control of Renal Glutamine Metabolism and NH_4^+ Excretion

There are several adaptive physiological controls over the production and tubular handling of NH_4^+. First, the renal metabolism of glutamine is subject to physiological control by extracellular pH. A decrease in plasma pH stimulates renal glutamine oxidation, whereas an increase does just the opposite.[12] (The control point is the enzyme glutaminase and/or altered transport into mitochondria, but the precise signal connecting pH changes to these events is unknown.) Thus, an acidosis, by stimulating renal glutamine oxidation, causes the kidneys to contribute more new

[12] Acidosis also causes a marked increase in hepatic glutamine synthesis, thereby supplying to the kidneys the additional glutamine required for increased renal glutamine metabolism (see Welbourne in Suggested Readings).

Table 9-2 Homeostatic Control of the Processes that Determine Renal Compensations for Acid-Base Disturbances

1. Phosphate reabsorption is inhibited during acidosis, thereby providing more luminal buffer to combine with secreted hydrogen ions.
2. Glutamine metabolism and NH_4^+ excretion are increased during acidosis and decreased during alkalosis. The signal is unknown.
3. Tubular hydrogen-ion secretion is
   a. Increased by the increased blood P_{CO_2} of respiratory acidosis and decreased by the decreased P_{CO_2} of respiratory alkalosis.
   b. Increased, independently of changes in P_{CO_2}, by the local effects of decreased extracellular pH on the tubules; the opposite is true for increased extracellular pH.
   c. Increased by the increased plasma aldosterone that occurs in metabolic acidosis.
4. Bicarbonate secretion by the cortical collecting duct is increased in alkalosis. The signal is unknown.

bicarbonate to the blood, thereby counteracting the acidosis. This pH responsiveness increases over the first few days of an acidosis and allows the glutamine-NH_4^+ mechanism for new bicarbonate generation to become the preeminent renal process for opposing the acidosis. Conversely, an alkalosis inhibits glutamine metabolism, resulting in little or no renal contribution of new bicarbonate via this route.

In addition to this control of NH_4^+ *production* by pH, it is likely that one or more of the complex transport processes that lead to *excretion* of the produced NH_4^+ is also influenced adaptively by extracellular pH. Thus, it is probable that acidosis influences transport in ways that enhance excretion, whereas alkalosis does the opposite.

In conclusion, acidosis increases renal NH_4^+ synthesis and excretion, whereas alkalosis does the opposite. This explains the spectrum of changes in NH_4^+ excretion summarized in the previous section.

Control of Tubular Hydrogen-Ion Secretion

Since tubular hydrogen-ion secretion is required for both bicarbonate reabsorption and the new bicarbonate production associated with titratable acid formation, the rate of hydrogen-ion secretion is a critical regulated variable. Before describing several of the physiological controls of hydrogen-ion secretion, let us review what "ought" to happen to produce the "desired" renal compensation (look again at the three data sets of the previous section).

When acid-base status is normal, the tubules should secrete enough hydrogen ion to achieve complete reabsorption of virtually all filtered bicarbonate and have enough left over to form some titratable acid, thereby contributing new bicarbonate to the blood (recall that our diet usually produces new hydrogen ions, which must be covered by the kidney's new bicarbonate). During alkalosis, tubular secretion should be too low to achieve complete reabsorption of filtered bicarbonate so that bicarbonate can be lost in the urine; no titratable acid is formed because there are no secreted hydrogen ions available to combine with nonbicarbonate buffers and no new bicarbonate is contributed to the blood. During acidosis, tubular hydrogen-ion secretion should be high enough to reabsorb all filtered bicarbonate and have enough hydrogen ions left to form large quantities of titratable acid, thereby contributing large quantities of new bicarbonate to the blood.

What, then, are the signals that influence tubular hydrogen-ion secretion? The best studied has been P_{CO_2}, an increase in this variable causing an increased hydrogen-ion secretion, and a decrease causing a decrease. There are no nerves or hormones mediating this response. Rather, the renal tubular cells respond to the P_{CO_2} of the blood perfusing them. An increased P_{CO_2} of arterial blood, as occurs during respiratory acidosis, causes an equivalent increase in P_{CO_2} within the tubular cells. This result causes, by mass action, elevated intracellular hydrogen-ion concentration, and it is this change that, via a sequence of intracellular events, stimulates the rate of hydrogen-ion secretion. In other words, the stimulus for hydrogen-ion secretion is not the P_{CO_2} per se but rather the decreased intracellular pH it induces.[13]

A second type of signal that influences hydrogen-ion secretion in a homeostatic manner is a change in extracellular pH unrelated to P_{CO_2}. The generalization is that decreased extracellular pH stimulates hydrogen-ion secretion, whereas increased extracellular pH does the opposite. The tubular segment involved and precise nature of the signal remain uncertain.

It must be reemphasized that the influence just described—extracellular pH—acts locally, no nerves or hormones being involved. In addition to this local response to altered pH, however, there is also a *reflex* component to the normal tubular response to metabolic acidosis. Renin secretion is stimulated during metabolic acidosis, and the resulting increase in plasma aldosterone causes an increase in hydrogen-ion secretion by the collecting-duct system. This action of aldosterone, not previously mentioned in the book, is distinct from this hormone's actions on sodium and potassium transport (Table 9-3), and the mechanism is unknown.[14] Thus, aldosterone participates in the homeostatic response to metabolic acidosis. The effect is probably small compared to the simultaneously occuring local stimulation of hydrogen-ion secretion by the extracellular pH, but we shall see in a subsequent section that it can become very important in pathophysiological situations.

---

[13] The nephron segment(s) involved and mechanisms remain controversial (see Al-Awqati in Suggested Readings). For example, it is likely that the decreased intracellular pH induces the insertion of H-ATPase pumps in the luminal membrane of at least one collecting-duct segment.

[14] The nephron segment stimulated is the outer medullary collecting duct. Aldosterone also stimulates NH_4^+ production and excretion.

Table 9-3   Summary of Aldosterone's Major Renal Actions

1. Stimulates sodium reabsorption
2. Stimulates potassium secretion
3. Stimulates hydrogen-ion secretion

Let us now apply the material covered so far to the specific categories of acid-base disorders.

Specific Categories of Acid-Base Disorders

Renal Compensation for Respiratory Acidosis and Alkalosis   For reference, we shall present the basic equations again. (CO_2 rather than H_2CO_3 can be used in the second equation because their concentrations are always in direct proportion to one another.)

$$H_2O + CO_2 \rightleftharpoons H_2CO_3 \rightleftharpoons H^+ + HCO_3^-$$

$$H^+ = K \, (CO_2/HCO_3^-)$$

In chronic pulmonary insufficiency, carbon dioxide is retained, and the resulting increase in arterial P_{CO_2} drives, by mass action, the formation of more H^+, with a resulting acidosis. It should be clear from the second equation that the pH could be restored to normal if the bicarbonate could be elevated to the same degree as the P_{CO_2}.[15]
It is the kidneys' job to cause this bicarbonate increase by contributing new bicarbonate to the blood. This occurs because (1) NH_4^+ production and excretion are increased by the acidosis, and (2) the increased P_{CO_2} stimulates renal-tubular hydrogen-ion secretion so that all filtered bicarbonate is reabsorbed and much secreted hydrogen-ion is left over for the formation of titratable acid, with its associated contribution of new bicarbonate to the blood. This latter process continues until a new steady state is reached. The renal compensation is not usually perfect; i.e., when

---

[15] There is, of course, an automatic increase, by mass action, in bicarbonate concentration solely as a result of the reaction being driven to the right by the elevated P_{CO_2}, but this is not nearly to the same degree, percentage-wise, as the rise in P_{CO_2}. If we transpose the second equation, we can see why mass action alone does not lead to proportionate increases of bicarbonate and carbon dioxide when P_{CO_2} increases.

$$[H^+] \, [HCO_3^-] = K[CO_2]$$

This form of the equation emphasizes that a rise in carbon dioxide causes a proportionate rise in the *product* $[H^+] \, [HCO_3^-]$. Since hydrogen-ion concentration increases, bicarbonate concentration cannot increase as much as carbon dioxide does or else the $[H^+] \, [HCO_3^-]$ product would rise more than proportionally. Plug in some real numbers and convince yourself that this is true.

the steady state is reached, the plasma bicarbonate is not elevated to quite the same degree as is the P_{CO_2}. Consequently, blood pH is not completely returned to normal.

The sequence of events in response to respiratory alkalosis is just the opposite. Respiratory alkalosis is the result of hyperventilation, in which the person transiently eliminates carbon dioxide faster than it is produced, thereby lowering his or her arterial P_{CO_2} and raising pH. The decreased P_{CO_2} reduces tubular hydrogen-ion secretion so that bicarbonate reabsorption is not complete. Bicarbonate is, therefore, lost from the body, and the loss results in decreased plasma bicarbonate and a return of plasma pH toward normal.

Renal Compensation for Metabolic Acidosis and Alkalosis Any acid-base disturbance not caused by a primary change in P_{CO_2} is termed *metabolic*. The primary cause of metabolic acidosis is either the addition to the body (by ingestion, infusion, or production) of increased amounts of any acid other than carbonic acid or, alternatively, the loss from the body of bicarbonate (as in diarrhea). Inspection of the equations reveals that either loss of bicarbonate or addition of hydrogen ions will lower both the plasma pH and the plasma bicarbonate concentration. The kidneys' compensation is to raise the plasma bicarbonate concentration back toward normal, thereby returning pH toward normal. To do this, the kidneys must reabsorb all the filtered bicarbonate and contribute new bicarbonate through the formation of ammonium and titratable acid. This is precisely what normal kidneys do, and the urines excreted in respiratory and metabolic acidosis are indistinguishable in these respects.

The increased NH_4^+ production and excretion triggered by the acidosis is predictable from previous sections, but the total reabsorption of bicarbonate and large formation of titratable acid requires more comment because the two major signals for hydrogen-ion secretion described in the previous section—P_{CO_2} and extracelluallar pH—are in opposed directions. The decreased extracellular pH (as well as the increased aldosterone reflexly triggered by it) is appropriately signaling for an increased hydrogen-ion secretion, but what about the P_{CO_2}? This variable is usually *decreased* in metabolic acidosis because, as the arterial pH falls as a result of whatever is causing the metabolic acidosis, pulmonary ventilation is reflexly stimulated. This is, of course, the respiratory compensation for the acidosis, and its effect is to reduce arterial P_{CO_2}. Therefore, because renal-tubular cell pH is rapidly altered by changes in P_{CO_2}, renal-tubular cell pH is likely to be *increased* in the early stages of metabolic acidosis.[16]

---

[16] In patients with chronic metabolic acidosis, it is likely that intracellular pH returns to normal or actually decreases, despite a continued decrease in P_{CO_2}, probably because of altered basolateral-membrane transport of hydrogen ion.

How, then, can the kidneys manage fully to perform their compensatory function with the decreased P_{CO_2} opposing the increased hydrogen-ion secretion being signalled for by the low extracellular pH? This apparent paradox is resolved when one recalls that in metabolic acidosis the plasma bicarbonate is lower than normal. Therefore, the mass of bicarbonate filtered (GFR $\times$ $P_{HCO_3^-}$) is reduced proportionally to the decreased plasma bicarbonate, and less hydrogen ion needs to be secreted to accomplish total reabsorption of the filtered bicarbonate. Accordingly, even with an unchanged or decreased total hydrogen-ion secretion rate, there is still considerable hydrogen ion available after the bicarbonate has been completely reabsorbed to form large amounts of titratable acid, thereby contributing new bicarbonate to the plasma. For example, compare the data for a person with metabolic acidosis with those for a normal person:

	Normal	Metabolic acidosis
Plasma HCO_3^-	24 mmol/L	12 mmol/L
GFR	180 L/day	180 L/day
Filtered HCO_3^-	4320 mmol/day	2160 mmol/day
1 Reabsorbed HCO_3^-	4315 mmol/day	2160 mmol/day
2 Titratable acid	20 mmol/day	80 mmol/day
3 Total H^+ secreted [1 + 2]	4335 mmol/day	2240 mmol/day

The situation in metabolic alkalosis is just the opposite. Despite a normal or increased rate of hydrogen-ion secretion secondary to a reflexly elevated P_{CO_2}, the load of filtered bicarbonate is so great that much bicarbonate escapes reabsorption. Also, as we have seen, bicarbonate secretion occurs in the cortical collecting duct in metabolic alkalosis. Overall, then, plasma bicarbonate is decreased, and pH decreases toward normal.[17]

FACTORS CAUSING THE KIDNEYS TO GENERATE OR MAINTAIN A METABOLIC ALKALOSIS

The previous sections described the mechanisms by which NH_4^+ production and hydrogen-ion secretion are controlled to achieve acid-base homeostasis. We now describe how factors *not* designed to maintain a constant pH can also influence these processes. In other words, just as is

---

[17] Recent evidence suggests that this description of how the kidney manages to increase bicarbonate excretion despite the stimulus to hydrogen-ion secretion exerted by a reflexly elevated P_{CO_2} may not fully apply to chronic situations. (See Madias et al. in Suggested Readings.)

true for potassium, hydrogen-ion balance has its own distinct homeostatic controls, but it is also at the mercy of other interacting factors. The most important of these are extracellular volume contraction, chloride depletion, and the combination of aldosterone excess and potassium depletion. The key point in all these situations is oversecretion of hydrogen-ion (and, sometimes, NH_4^+, as well), producing one of two general results: (1) The kidneys may generate a metabolic alkalosis, or (2) the kidneys may not generate a metabolic alkalosis but may fail to do their usual job of compensating for an already existing metabolic alkalosis.

Influence of Extracellular Volume Contraction

The presence of extracellular volume contraction because of salt depletion interferes with the ability of the kidneys to compensate for a metabolic alkalosis. In metabolic alkalosis, the plasma bicarbonate is elevated, either because of the addition of bicarbonate to the body or because of the loss of hydrogen ion from it. The normal renal compensation should be to set hydrogen-ion secretion at a level that fails to achieve complete bicarbonate reabsorption and thereby allows the excess bicarbonate to be excreted. But the presence of the extracellular volume contraction not only stimulates sodium reabsorption but also stimulates hydrogen-ion secretion. As described earlier, aldosterone stimulates hydrogen-ion secretion, and the elevated aldosterone in extracellular volume contraction probably accounts for a portion of the oversecretion of hydrogen ion. However, other, as yet unidentified, factors seem to be of greater importance. Whatever the mechanism, the net result is that all the filtered bicarbonate is reabsorbed so that the already elevated plasma bicarbonate associated with the preexisting metabolic alkalosis is locked in, and the plasma pH remains unchanged. The urine, instead of being alkaline, as it should be when the kidneys are normally compensating for a metabolic alkalosis, is somewhat acid.

Influence of Chloride Depletion

We referred to extracellular volume contraction in the previous section without distinguishing between sodium and chloride losses as the cause because loss of either of these ions will lead to extracellular volume contraction. Now, however, we must emphasize that specific chloride depletion, in a manner independent of and in addition to extracellular volume contraction, helps maintain metabolic alkalosis by stimulating hydrogen-ion secretion. The mechanisms for the specific chloride-depletion effect remain unclear, but the phenomenon has considerable clinical importance because many situations (vomiting, for example) are associated with both metabolic alkalosis and chloride depletion.

Influence of Aldosterone Excess and Potassium Depletion

As noted several times, aldosterone stimulates hydrogen-ion secretion (and NH_4^+ production), although the effect is relatively modest. Now we shall see that when to this effect is added another event—potassium depletion—a marked increase in hydrogen-ion secretion is induced.

Potassium depletion, by itself, also tends to stimulate tubular hydrogen-ion secretion (and ammonium production). Presumably, potassium depletion of renal-tubular cells causes a decrease in renal-cell pH (because of the reciprocal relations between cell pH and potassium described in the previous chapter), and it is this decrease that stimulates hydrogen-ion secretion. For many years, it has been argued whether or not potassium depletion, *by itself,* can stimulate tubular hydrogen-ion secretion enough to alter significantly the renal contribution to acid-base balance. Most evidence now indicates that this may sometimes be the case, but only when the degree of potassium depletion is extremely severe.[18]

Now we come to the critical point. The combination of potassium depletion of even moderate degree and high levels of aldosterone acts synergistically to stimulate tubular hydrogen-ion secretion markedly. As a result, the renal tubules not only reabsorb all filtered bicarbonate but also contribute inappropriately large amounts of new bicarbonate to the body, thereby causing the development of metabolic alkalosis. Note that there may have been nothing wrong with the acid-base balance to start with: The alkalosis is actually generated by the kidneys themselves. Of course, if alkalosis were already present because of some other cause, this high-aldosterone/potassium-depletion combination would not only prevent the kidneys from compensating but also make the alkalosis worse.

This phenomenon is important because the combination of a markedly elevated aldosterone and potassium depletion occurs in a variety of clinical situations. One reason for their coexistence is that the former can cause the latter. Recall from Chap. 8 that aldosterone stimulates potassium secretion; therefore, a very high level of aldosterone may cause potassium depletion via the urine. The potassium depletion and high aldosterone then act together to induce the kidneys to generate a metabolic alkalosis. A good example is the patient with primary hypersection of aldosterone because of an adrenal tumor (Fig. 9-5).

A much more common situation in which a high plasma-aldosterone

---

[18] One reason for the failure of potassium depletion by itself to produce a significant excess of hydrogen-ion secretion is that potassium depletion inhibits secretion of aldosterone (as described in Chap. 8). Accordingly, the stimulatory effect aldosterone tonically exerts on hydrogen-ion secretion is lost, and this loss offsets the stimulatory effect exerted by potassium depletion.

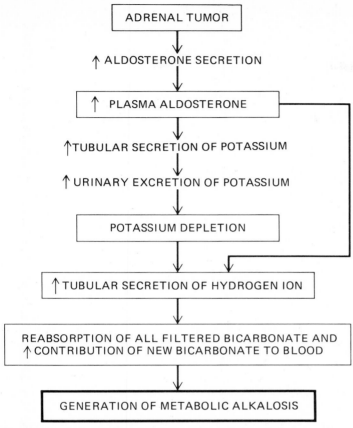

Figure 9-5 Pathway for generation of metabolic alkalosis in a patient with primary hyperaldosteronism.

concentration and potassium depletion coexist is the extensive use of diuretic drugs (Fig. 9-6). This combination can then act to generate a metabolic alkalosis. Note also that the person in this example is triply in trouble: As described in the previous sections, extracellular-volume contraction per se, via a mechanism unrelated to aldosterone, stimulates reabsorption of bicarbonate. This helps to maintain the alkalosis once the high-aldosterone/potassium-depletion combination has generated it. Indeed, if the diuretics have also produced chloride depletion in addition to the extracellular volume contraction, the person will be quadruply in trouble because chloride depletion, as described above, causes excessive secretion of hydrogen ion.

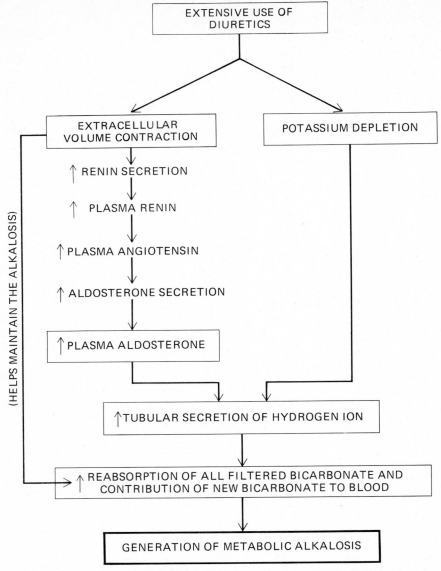

Figure 9-6   Pathway by which overuse of diuretics leads to a metabolic alkalosis. Note that the extracellular volume contraction, via a nonaldosterone mechanism, helps to maintain the alkalosis once it has been generated. If the diuretics have also caused chloride depletion, this too will contribute to the maintenance of the metabolic alkalosis.

Study questions: 64 to 72

10

REGULATION OF CALCIUM AND PHOSPHATE BALANCE

OBJECTIVES

The student understands the regulation of calcium balance and extracellular concentration.

1 States the normal plasma calcium concentration and the percentage that is protein-bound; states the effect of pH on the free and bound fractions
2 Describes the gastrointestinal handling of calcium
3 Describes the basic renal handling of calcium; states the effects of changes in sodium intake and of metabolic acidosis on calcium excretion
4 States the percentage of total-body calcium in bone
5 Lists the effects of parathyroid hormone and their adaptive value
6 Describes the control of secretion of parathyroid hormone
7 Describes the sequence of reactions leading from 7-dehydrocholesterol to 1,25-$(OH)_2D_3$; states the major control over the 1-hydroxylation step
8 Lists the effects of 1,25-$(OH)_2D_3$
9 Defines calcitonin and states its suggested role in calcium regulation
10 Predicts changes in plasma and urinary calcium and phosphate in patients with hyperparathyroidism or with 1,25-$(OH)_2D_3$ deficiency
11 States the effects of cortisol and growth hormone on calcium balance

The student understands the renal regulation of phosphate balance.

1 Describes the renal handling of phosphate
2 States two mechanisms that cause increased urinary phosphate excretion when dietary phosphate is elevated
3 States the effects of parathyroid hormone and 1,25-$(OH)_2D_3$ on tubular reabsorption of phosphate

Extracellular calcium concentration is normally maintained within very narrow limits, the requirement for precise regulation stemming primarily from the profound effects of calcium on neuromuscular excitability. A low calcium concentration increases the excitability of nerve and muscle cell membranes so that patients with diseases in which low calcium occurs suffer from **hypocalcemic tetany,** characterized by skeletal muscle spasms, which can be severe enough to cause death by asphyxia. Hypercalcemia is dangerous, too, because it causes cardiac arrhythmias as well as depressed neuromuscular excitability. All these effects reflect calcium's ability to bind to plasma-membrane proteins that function as ion channels, altering their open or closed state. This effect of calcium on membranes is totally distinct from its role as an excitation-contraction coupler.

It is important to recognize that the plasma calcium (normally 5 meq/L or 2.5 mmol/L) exists in three general forms in approximately the following proportions: (1) 45 percent is in the ionized (Ca^{2+}) form, the only biologically active form in nerve, muscle, and other target organs; (2) 15 percent is complexed to anions with relatively low molecular weights, such as citrate and phosphate; (3) 40 percent is reversibly bound to plasma proteins. One of the most important influences on protein binding is the plasma pH. An increase in pH causes increased calcium binding because the decreased acidity converts more of the protein to the anionic form; i.e., it exposes additional negatively charged binding sites. Thus, a patient with alkalosis is susceptible to tetany, whereas a patient with acidosis will not manifest tetany at levels of total plasma calcium low enough to cause symptoms in normal people.

EFFECTOR SITES FOR CALCIUM HOMEOSTASIS

Normally, the body remains in stable calcium balance; i.e., the amount of ingested calcium is equal to the calcium lost in urine, feces, and sweat combined. However, in contrast to the situation for the other ions described in this book, the major variable homeostatically controlled to achieve this balance is not the rate of urinary excretion but rather the rate of gastrointestinal absorption.

Earlier chapters on ion and water homeostasis were concerned almost entirely with the *renal* handling of these substances. It was possible to do so for several reasons: (1) Although internal exchanges (between extracellular fluid, on the one hand, and bone and cells, on the other) are of some importance for these substances, the major homeostatic controls act via the kidneys. (2) Intestinal absorption of these substances approximates 100 percent under normal circumstances and is not a major controlled variable. Neither of these statements holds true for calcium homeostasis. Accordingly, this section must deal not only with the renal handling of calcium but also with the other two major effector sites for calcium homeostasis—bone and the gastrointestinal tract.

Gastrointestinal Tract

Under normal conditions a considerable amount of ingested calcium is not absorbed from the intestine and simply leaves the body along with the feces. Indeed, fecal calcium excretion can exceed calcium ingestion since calcium is also secreted into the intestinal lumen. Accordingly, control of the active transport system that moves calcium from intestinal lumen to blood can result in large increases or decreases in net calcium absorption. Control of this absorptive process is the major means for homeostatically regulating total-body calcium balance.

Kidneys

The kidneys handle calcium by filtration and reabsorption. Only about 60 percent of the plasma calcium is filterable, the remainder being protein-bound. Reabsorption[1] occurs throughout the nephron, with the exception of the descending limb of Henle's loop, and its quantitative pattern is similar to that of sodium: About 60 percent of reabsorption occurs proximally and the remainder in the ascending limb of Henle's loop, distal convoluted tubule, and collecting ducts. Reabsorption normally approximates 98 to 99 percent, the 1 to 2 percent escaping reabsorption generally being equal to the normal net addition of new calcium to the body via the gastrointestinal tract. Thus, just as was true for the other ions discussed in this book, the kidneys help maintain a constant balance of total-body calcium by matching output to intake; when intake is altered, the rate of excretion is homeostatically altered. However, the kidneys respond to changes in dietary calcium much less than they do to changes in sodium, water, or potassium. For example, it has been estimated that only about 5 percent of an increment in dietary calcium appears in the urine because most of the dietary increment fails to be absorbed from the gastrointestinal tract. At the other end of the spectrum, when dietary intake of calcium is reduced to extremely low levels, there is a slow reduction of urinary calcium, but some continues to appear in the urine for weeks.

How do the renal homeostatic mechanisms operate? Since calcium is filtered and reabsorbed, but not secreted,

$$\text{Ca excretion} = \text{Ca filtered} - \text{Ca reabsorbed}$$

Accordingly, excretion can be altered homeostatically by changing either the filtered load or the rate of reabsorption. Both occur. For example, what happens when a person increases his or her calcium intake? Tran-

---

[1] The cellular mechanisms of calcium reabsorption vary in different segments and are still not clearly worked out (see Suki and Rouse in Suggested Readings).

siently, intake exceeds output, positive calcium balance ensues, and plasma calcium concentration increases. This in itself increases the filtered mass of calcium and increases excretion. Simultaneously, as we shall see, the increased plasma calcium triggers hormonal changes that cause a diminished reabsorption. The net result of these responses is increased calcium excretion.

A bewildering array of factors *not* designed to maintain calcium homeostasis can also influence urinary calcium excretion, mainly by stimulating or inhibiting tubular reabsorption. These include a large number of hormones, ions, acid-base disturbances, and drugs (see Suki in Suggested Readings). One of the most important of them is sodium. Under many circumstances, changes in calcium excretion can be induced simply by administering or withholding salt. (This fact is used clinically when one wishes to increase or decrease the amount of calcium in the body.) Indeed, changes in dietary sodium may be more effective in altering urinary calcium excretion than are changes in dietary calcium. Clearly, there is some kind of coupling between sodium reabsorption and calcium reabsorption, at least in the proximal tubule and loop of Henle. In contrast, these two ions can be dissociated in the more distal nephron segments since their major hormonal controls—aldosterone (sodium) and parathyroid hormone (calcium)—stimulate reabsorption at these sites only of one ion without affecting the other.[2]

A second very important factor that influences tubular calcium reabsorption but is not designed to maintain calcium homeostatis is chronic metabolic acidosis. The mechanism is not known, but acidosis markedly inhibits calcium reabsorption and, hence, causes increased calcium excretion. Chronic metabolic alkalosis tends to do just the opposite—enhance calcium reabsorption and reduce excretion.

Bone

The activities of the gastrointestinal tract and the kidneys determine the net intake and output of calcium for the entire body and, thereby, the overall state of calcium balance. In contrast, interchanges of calcium between extracellular fluid and bone do not alter total-body balance but, rather, the distribution of calcium within the body. Approximately 99 percent of the total-body calcium is contained in bone, which is basically a collagen-protein framework on which calcium phosphate (and other minerals) are deposited in a crystal structure known as **hydroxyapatite.** Bone is not a dead, fixed tissue; rather, it is cellular and well supplied with blood. Most important, it is continuously broken down (resorbed) and

[2] An interesting indication of the differences in reabsorption of these two ions in the distal convoluted tubule is the fact that thiazide diuretics inhibit distal sodium reabsorption but facilitate distal calcium reabsorption. In contrast, diuretics that act mainly in the proximal tubule and/or loop of Henle inhibit reabsorption of both ions.

simultaneously re-formed under the influence of the bone cells. Thus, bone provides a huge potential source or sink for the withdrawal or deposit of calcium from extracellular fluid. We shall see that several hormones exert important effects on the deposition or resorption of bone calcium.

HORMONAL CONTROL OF EFFECTOR SITES

Parathyroid Hormone

All three of the effector sites described above are subject to direct or indirect control by a polypeptide hormone called **parathyroid hormone,** produced by the **parathyroid glands.** Parathyroid-hormone production is controlled directly by the calcium concentration of the extracellular fluid bathing the cells of these glands. Decreased plasma calcium concentration stimulates parathyroid-hormone production and release, and increased plasma concentration does just the opposite. Extracellular calcium concentration acts directly on the parathyroids without any intermediary hormones or nerves.

Parathyroid hormone exerts at least four distinct effects on calcium homeostasis (Figs. 10-1 and 10-2):

1   It increases the movement of calcium from bone into extracellular fluid by stimulating bone resorption. In this manner the immense store of calcium contained in bone is made available for the regulation of extracellular calcium concentration.

2   It stimulates the activation of vitamin D (see below), and this hormone then increases intestinal absorption of calcium.

3   It increases renal-tubular calcium reabsorption, by an action on the distal convoluted tubule, and thus decreases urinary calcium excretion.

4   It reduces the proximal-tubular reabsorption of phosphate, thereby raising urinary phosphate excretion and lowering extracellular phosphate concentration.

The adaptive value of the first three effects should be obvious: They all result in a higher extracellular calcium concentration and thus compensate for the lower concentration that originally stimulated parathyroid-hormone production. The adaptive value of the fourth effect requires further explanation, as follows.

When parathyroid hormone induces bone resorption, both calcium and phosphate are released. Similarly, vitamin D enhances the intestinal absorption of both calcium and phosphate. Accordingly, while the low calcium, which triggered the increase in parathyroid hormone, is being

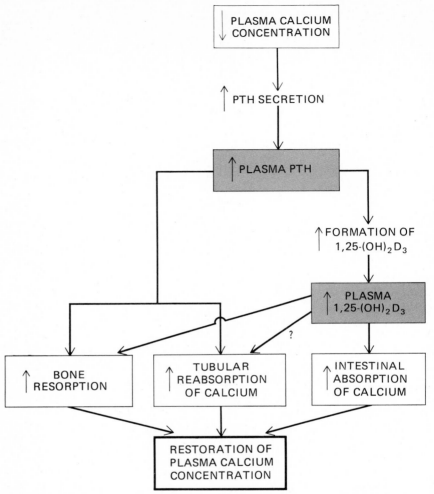

Figure 10-1 Hormonally mediated compensatory response to reduced plasma calcium concentration. PTH = parathyroid hormone. The effects of PTH and $1,25\text{-}(OH)_2D_3$ on phosphate are not shown in the figure (see text and Fig. 10-2).

homeostatically compensated for, the plasma phosphate would tend to be raised above normal. However, plasma phosphate does not actually increase because of the parathyroid hormone's inhibition of tubular phosphate reabsorption. Indeed, so potent is this effect that plasma phosphate may actually decrease when parathyroid-hormone levels are elevated. (This reduction in phosphate is adaptive in that it facilitates further bone resorption because of local interactions between calcium and phosphate.)

In contrast to the state described above, an increase in extracellular calcium concentration reduces parathyroid-hormone production and, thereby, produces increased urinary and fecal calcium loss and net movement of calcium from extracellular fluid into bone.

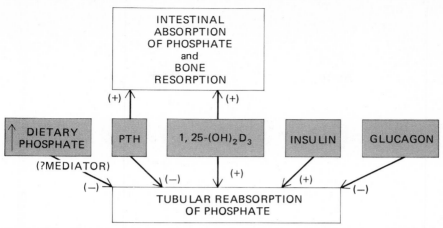

Figure 10-2 Effects of hormones and dietary phosphate on phosphate movements. (+) denotes a stimulation, and (−) an inhibition. Moreover, each (+) will tend to raise plasma phosphate concentration, whereas each (−) will tend to lower it.

Parathyroid hormone has other functions in the body, but the four effects discussed constitute the major mechanisms by which it integrates various organs and tissues in the regulation of extracellular calcium concentration.[3]

Hyperparathyroidism, resulting from a primary defect in the parathyroid glands (e.g., a hormone-secreting tumor), well illustrates the actions of parathyroid hormone. The excess hormone causes enhanced bone resorption, leading to bone thinning and the formation of completely calcium-free areas or cysts. Plasma calcium increases and plasma phosphate decreases; the latter is caused by increased urinary phosphate excretion. The increased plasma calcium is deposited in various body tissues, including the kidneys, where stones are formed. A seeming paradox is that urinary calcium excretion is increased despite the fact that tubular calcium reabsorption is enhanced by parathyroid hormone. The explanation is that because of the elevated plasma calcium induced by the nonrenal effects of parathyriod hormone, the filtered load of calcium increases even more than does the reabsorptive rate. This result nicely illustrates the necessity of taking both filtration and reabsorption into account when analyzing excretory changes of any substance.

[3] Another candidate to join these four was described in Chap. 9—parathyroid hormone's inhibition of proximal-tubular hydrogen-ion secretion and, thereby, bicarbonate reabsorption. The result of this effect is increased extracellular fluid hydrogen-ion concentration (acidosis), which is known to displace calcium from plasma protein (as described above) and from bone. Thus, free plasma calcium concentration rises. Whether this effect of parathyroid hormone is really important at physiological plasma levels of the hormone is still not settled. It is likely that parathyroid hormone can induce a metabolic acidosis in ways other than its inhibition of tubular hydrogen-ion secretion. (See Hulter in Suggested Readings for Chap. 9.)

1,25-Dihydroxyvitamin D_3

The term **vitamin D** denotes a group of closely related sterols. One of these compounds, called **vitamin D_3** (or cholecalciferol), is formed by the action of ultraviolet radiation on 7-dehydrocholesterol in the skin. A second source of vitamin D is that ingested in food, specifically in plants. Because of clothing and decreased out-of-doors living, people are often dependent on this dietary source. The form of vitamin D found naturally in food differs only trivially in structure from vitamin D_3, and no distinction will be made between them in the subsequent description.

Vitamin D_3 is inactive and must undergo metabolic changes within the body before it can influence its target cells. It enters the blood and is hydroxylated in the 25 position by the liver and then in the 1 position by the kidneys. The end result is the active form of vitamin D—**1,25-dihydroxyvitamin D_3**, abbreviated **1,25-$(OH)_2D_3$**. From this description, it should be evident that 1,25-$(OH)_2D_3$ is actually a hormone, not a vitamin, since it is made in the body.

The major action of 1,25-$(OH)_2D_3$ is to stimulate active absorption of calcium (and phosphate) by the intestine. Thus, the major event in vitamin D deficiency is decreased gut calcium absorption, resulting in decreased plasma calcium. In children, the newly formed bone protein matrix fails to be calcified normally because of the low plasma calcium, leading to the disease **rickets.**

In addition to its effect on intestinal calcium absorption, 1,25-$(OH)_2D_3$ also significantly enhances bone resorption. The mechanism underlying this effect is unclear but may involve a facilitation by 1,25-$(OH)_2D_3$ of the bone resorption effect exerted by parathyroid hormone. Finally, 1,25-$(OH)_2D_3$ can also stimulate the renal-tubular reabsorption of calcium (and phosphate), but whether this effect is significant physiologically remains unsettled.

The blood concentration of 1,25-$(OH)_2D_3$ is subject to physiological control. The major control point is the second hydroxylation step, the one that occurs in the kidneys. This step is stimulated by parathyroid hormone, a phenomenon that is highly adaptive because it provides a mechanism for simultaneously altering the levels of these hormones in the same direction. Thus, a low plasma-calcium concentration stimulates the secretion of parathyroid hormone, which in turn enhances the production of 1,25-$(OH)_2D_3$, and both hormones contribute to the restoration of the plasma calcium to normal (Fig. 10-1).[4]

[4] Parathyroid hormone is not the only modulator of 1,25-$(OH)_2D_3$ formation. Phosphate is another important one, decreased plasma phosphate stimulating formation. This is adaptive in terms of phosphate homeostasis: Decreased phosphate stimulates formation of 1,25-$(OH)_2D_3$, which then enhances phosphate absorption from the gut (and possibly, its reabsorption by the renal tubules), with a resulting compensatory increase in plasma phosphate. Many other possible inputs are presently being studied. For example, it is likely that estrogen and prolactin also stimulate formation of 1,25-$(OH)_2D_3$. This would be adaptive in increasing gut absorption of calcium and phosphate during pregnancy.

Calcitonin

Yet a third hormone, calcitonin, has significant effects on plasma calcium. **Calcitonin** is a peptide hormone secreted by cells within the thyroid gland that surround, but are completely distinct from, the thyroid follicles. The calcitonin-secreting cells are called, therefore, **parafollicular cells.** Calcitonin can lower plasma calcium, primarily by inhibiting bone resorption. Its secretion is controlled, in part, directly by the calcium concentration of the plasma supplying the thyroid gland; increased calcium causes increased calcitonin secretion. Thus, this system has been suspected of constituting another feedback control over plasma calcium concentration. However, its overall contribution to calcium homeostasis is very minor compared with that of parathyroid hormone and $1,25\text{-}(OH)_2D_3$. Indeed, thyroidectomized persons with no detectable plasma calcitonin have no significant alteration in their plasma calcium concentration. Accordingly, emphasis has shifted away from calcitonin as a regulator of plasma calcium and toward its possible roles in regulating other physiological activities.[5]

Other Hormones

Parathyroid hormone and $1,25\text{-}(OH)_2D_3$ are the major hormones that participate in homeostatic responses to changes in calcium balance. However, several other hormones do influence calcium, so that changes in their rates of secretion can produce calcium imbalances. Thus, high levels of cortisol can induce negative calcium balance by depressing gut absorption of calcium while increasing its renal excretion. Growth hormone also increases urinary calcium excretion, but it simultaneously increases gut absorption; the net effect of these counterbalancing influences of growth hormone is usually a positive calcium balance.

OVERVIEW OF RENAL PHOSPHATE HANDLING

The renal handling of phosphate has been mentioned several times in this chapter and elsewhere in the book but almost always in the context of other topics, such as sodium reabsorption or urine acidification. This section reviews certain key aspects of renal phosphate handling since control of urinary phosphate excretion is a major pathway for the homeostatic regulation of total-body phosphate balance.

Approximately 5 to 10 percent of plasma phosphate is protein-bound, so that 90 to 95 percent is filterable at the renal corpuscle. Normally, approximately 75 percent of this filtered phosphate is actively reabsorbed, mainly in the proximal tubule (in cotransport with sodium). There

---

[5] See Austin and Heath in Suggested Readings.

is probably also some small degree of phosphate reabsorption in sites beyond the proximal tubule. There is no conclusive evidence for significant tubular secretion of phosphate (although this remains controversial).

As with other substances handled by filtration and tubular reabsorption, the rate of phosphate excretion can be changed by altering the mass filtered per unit time and/or the mass reabsorbed per unit time. Because the reabsorptive T_m for phosphate is very close to the normal filtered load, even relatively small increases in plasma phosphate concentration (and, hence, filtered load) can produce relatively large increases in phosphate excretion. This occurs when plasma phosphate concentration increases as a result of increased dietary phosphate intake.

But changes is filtered load are not the major reason that phosphate excretion increases or decreases homeostatically in response to altered dietary intake. Tubular reabsorption also changes. A diet low in phosphate induces, over time, an increase in the rate of phosphate reabsorption (as well as an increase in the transport maximum for phosphate); a diet high in phosphate does just the opposite. These homeostatic adaptations are not due to changes in parathyroid hormone or $1,25\text{-}(OH)_2D_3$, and the pathways and mechanisms involved remain unknown.

As noted in Chap. 9, another physiological situation in which phosphate reabsorption is decreased is acidosis. Here, too, the mechanism for this adaptive response (it provides more buffer to form titratable acid) is not known.

To reiterate, changes in parathyroid hormone do not mediate the homeostatic association between dietary phosphate and tubular phosphate reabsorption, nor do they account for altered phosphate excretion in acidosis. Nevertheless, as we have seen, whenever parathyroid hormone is increased or decreased, tubular phosphate reabsorption is powerfully inhibited or stimulated, respectively. Other hormones, too, are known to alter phosphate reabsorption. For example, $1,25\text{-}(OH)_2D_3$ and insulin increase it, and glucagon decreases it. These are only a few of the many factors that can influence phosphate reabsorption and, hence, phosphate excretion and balance (Fig. 10-2).

Study questions: 71 to 73

STUDY QUESTIONS

As emphasized in the preface, these questions do not cover the material of this book systematically or comprehensively; that is the function of the objectives at the beginning of each chapter. Rather, these questions provide practice and additional feedback in certain areas, particularly those that commonly give some difficulty.

Q-1 The difference between superficial and juxtamedullary nephrons is that the former have their glomeruli in the cortex whereas the glomeruli of the latter arise in the medulla. True or false?

A-1 False. All glomeruli are in the cortex. See text for description.

Q-2 When a patient is given a drug that inhibits angiotensin-converting enzyme, there is little physiological effect because the decrement in angiotensin II is compensated for by the simultaneous rise in angiotensin I. True or false?

A-2 False. Angiotensin II is much more potent than angiotensin I.

Q-3 Substance T is present in the urine. Does this *prove* that it is filterable at the glomerulus?

A-3 No. It is a possibility, but there is another: Substance T may be secreted by the tubules.

Q-4 Substance V is not normally present in the urine. Does this *prove* that it is neither filtered nor secreted?

A-4 No. It is a possibility, but there is another: V may be filtered and/or secreted, but all the V entering the lumen via these routes may be completely reabsorbed.

Q-5 The concentration of calcium in Bowman's capsule is 3mM, whereas its plasma concentration is 5mM. How do you explain this?

A-5 Approximately 40 percent of the calcium in plasma is bound to proteins and so is not filterable.

Q-6 The concentration of glucose in plasma is 100 mg/100mL and the GFR is 125 mL/min. How much glucose is filtered per minute?

A-6 125 mg/min. The amount of *any* substance filtered per unit time is given by the product of the GFR and the filterable plasma concentration of the substance, in this case, 125 mL/min $\times$ 100 mg/100 mL.

Q-7 A protein has a molecular weight of 20,000 and a plasma concentration of 100 mg/L. The GFR is 100 L/day. How much of this protein is filtered per day?

191

A-7 No exact value can be calculated from these data because the concentration of the protein in the glomerular filtrate is not known. The molecular weight is high enough so that some "sieving" would occur but low enough so that the restriction would not be total.

Q-8 A drug is noted to cause a decrease in GFR. What might the drug be doing?

A-8
a Constricting glomerular mesangial cells and, hence, reducing K_f
b Lowering arterial pressure and, hence, P_{GC}
c Constricting the afferent arteriole and, hence, reducing P_{GC}
d Dilating the efferent arteriole and, hence, reducing P_{GC}
e Causing obstruction somewhere in the urinary system and, hence, increasing P_{BC}
f Increasing plasma albumin concentration and, hence, π_{GC}
g Decreasing the amount of blood flow to the kidneys, resulting in a steeper use of π_{GC} along the length of the glomerular capillaries

Q-9 A drug is noted to cause an increase in GFR with no change in net filtration pressure. What must the drug be doing?

A-9 It must be increasing K_f, i.e., changing the hydraulic permeability of the gomerular membranes and/or the surface area available for filtration.

Q-10 Substance O is filtered, reabsorbed, and secreted. If you were designing a system for increasing the renal excretion of substance O when its intake is high, what could you do?

A-10 There are three possibilities (either alone or in combination): Increase filtered substance O by increasing either GFR or plasma concentration of substance O; inhibit tubular reabsorption of substance O; enhance tubular secretion of substance O.

Q-11 There is a net movement of anionic phosphate across the luminal membrane into the tubular cells even though cytosolic phosphate concentration is higher than luminal and there is a cytosol-negative potential difference across the luminal membrane. Does this prove that the phosphate movement is driven by the direct input of energy from splitting ATP?

A-11 No. It proves that the movement is active, but it could be a secondary active transport (and, in fact, is).

Q-12 You are trying to measure the reabsorptive T_m for glucose in a patient. You plan to calculate glucose reabsorption $[(\text{GFR} \times P_G) - (U_G \times V)]$ as you raise plasma glucose stepwise by infusion. You stop the test when glucose first appears in the urine, assuming that the reabsorptive rate at this time equals the T_m. Is this correct?

A-12 No. Glucose starts to appear in the urine *before* the T_m for all nephrons has been reached. Therefore, if you had continued to raise plasma glucose, the reabsorptive rate would have increased some more. You can be certain the T_m has been reached only when the reabsorptive rate remains constant despite another increment in plasma glucose.

Q-13 The hospital lab reports that your patient's creatinine clearance is 120 g/
day.
This value is
a Normal
b Significantly below normal
c Nonsense

A-13 (c). Clearance units are volume per time, not mass per time.

Q-14 The following test results were obtained on specimens from a person over a
2-h period during infusion of inulin and PAH.

$$
\begin{aligned}
\text{Total urine vol} &= 0.14\text{L} \\
U_{In} &= 100 \text{ mg/100mL} \\
P_{In} &= 1 \text{ mg/100mL} \\
U_{urea} &= 220 \text{ mmol/L} \\
P_{urea} &= 5 \text{ mmol/L} \\
U_{PAH} &= 700 \text{ mg/mL} \\
P_{PAH} &= 2\text{mg/mL} \\
\text{Hematocrit} &= 0.40
\end{aligned}
$$

What are the clearances of inulin, urea, and PAH? What is the effective
renal plasma flow (ERPF)? What is the effective renal blood flow (ERBF)?
How much urea is reabsorbed? How much PAH is secreted (assuming no
PAH reabsorption and complete filterability of PAH)?

A-14

$$
\begin{aligned}
C_{In} &= \frac{U_{In}V}{P_{In}} \\
&= \frac{100 \text{ mg/100 mL} \times 0.14 \text{ L/2 h}}{1 \text{ mg/100 mL}} \\
&= 14.0 \text{ L/2 h; this is the GFR} \\
C_{urea} &= \frac{U_{urea}V}{P_{urea}} \\
&= \frac{220 \text{ mmol/L} \times 0.14 \text{ L/2 h}}{5 \text{ mmol/L}} \\
&= 6.16 \text{ L/2 h} \\
C_{PAH} &= \frac{U_{PAH}V}{P_{PAH}} \\
&= \frac{700 \text{ mg/mL} \times 0.14 \text{ L/2 h}}{2 \text{ mg/mL}} \\
&= 49.0 \text{ L/2 h}
\end{aligned}
$$

$$
\begin{aligned}
\text{ERPF} &= 49.0 \text{ L/2 h} \\
\text{ERBF} &= 81.7 \text{ L/2 h} \\
\text{Reabsorbed urea} &= \text{filtered urea} - \text{excreted urea} \\
&= (14.0 \text{ L/2 h} \times 5 \text{ mmol/L} \\
&\quad -(220 \text{ mmol/L} \times 0.14 \text{ L/2 h}) \\
&= 39.2 \text{ mmol/2 h}
\end{aligned}
$$

$$PAH \text{ secreted} = PAH \text{ excreted} - PAH \text{ filtered}$$
$$= (700 \text{ mg/mL} \times 0.14 \text{ L/2 h})$$
$$- (2 \text{ mg/mL} \times 14.0 \text{ L/2 h})$$
$$= 98.0 \text{ g/2 h} - 28.0 \text{ g/2 h}$$
$$= 70.0 \text{ g/2 h}$$

Q-15 In Q-14, you also obtained a sample of plasma from a renal vein. Its PAH concentration was 0.2 mg/mL. Now that you know that the renal venous plasma contains PAH, is the value you calculated for secreted PAH the secretory T_m for PAH?

A-15 No. There is always PAH in the renal venous plasma, mainly because some of the renal blood flow does not pass near proximal tubules. The way to do a PAH secretory T_m is to keep raising the systemic plasma PAH by infusion, and when the mass of PAH secreted (calculated just as you did in the problem) stops increasing with further increments in systemic plasma PAH, that mass is the T_m.

Q-16 An increase in the plasma concentration of inulin causes which of the following in the renal clearance of inulin?
  a Increase
  b Decrease
  c No change

A-16 c. $C_{In} = U_{In}V/P_{In}$. When P_{In} increases, there is no change in C_{In} because U_{In} rises an identical amount. In other words, the mass of inulin filtered and excreted increases, but the volume of plasma supplying this inulin, i.e., completely cleared of inulin, is unaltered.

Q-17 The clearance of substance A is less than that simultaneously determined for inulin. Give three possible explanations.

A-17 1. Substance A is a large molecule poorly filtered at the glomerulus.
  2. Substance A is bound, at least in part, to plasma protein.
  3. Substance A is reabsorbed.

Q-18 The clearance of substance B is greater than the simultaneously determined clearance for inulin. What is the only possible explanation for this?

A-18 Substance B is secreted by the tubules.

Q-19 List in order of decreasing renal clearance the following substances.
  Glucose
  Urea
  Sodium
  Inulin
  Creatinine
  PAH

A-19 PAH
  Creatinine
  Inulin

Urea
Sodium
Glucose

Q-20 The following test results were obtained during a clearance experiment.

$$U_{In} = 50 \text{ mg/L}$$
$$P_{In} = 1 \text{ mg/L}$$
$$V = 2 \text{ mL/min}$$
$$U_{Na} = 75 \text{ mM}$$
$$P_{Na} = 150 \text{ mM}$$

What is the fractional excretion (FE) of sodium?

A-20 0.01.

$$FE_{Na} = \frac{\text{mass Na excreted}}{\text{mass Na filtered}} = \frac{U_{Na}V}{GFR \times P_{Na}} = \frac{U_{Na}V}{C_{In} \times P_{Na}}$$
$$= \frac{75 \text{ mmol/L} \times 2 \text{ ml/min}}{100 \text{ ml/min} \times 150 \text{ mmol/L}}$$
$$= 0.01$$

This means that only 1 percent of the filtered sodium was excreted; i.e., 99 percent was reabsorbed.

Q-21 During a micropuncture experiment, a sample of tubular fluid (TF) was obtained from the end of the proximal tubule and its inulin concentration was found to be twice as high as the concentration in plasma, i.e., $TF_{In}/P_{In} = 2$. How much water was reabsorbed by the proximal tubule?

A-21 Fifty percent of the water that was originally filtered. Since inulin is neither reabsorbed nor secreted, its rise in concentration along the tubule is due entirely to water reabsorption and can, therefore, be used to calculate the extent of water reabsorption.

Q-22 If 50 percent of a person's nephrons were destroyed, which of the following compounds would be likely to show increased blood concentration?
  a Urea
  b Creatinine
  c Uric acid
  d Most amino acids
  e Glucose

A-22 a, b, c. These waste products are all normally excreted in large amounts; a decreased GFR would cause their plasma concentrations to increase until the filtered load was increased enough to reestablish normal excretion. In contrast, the reabsorption T_ms for glucose, amino acids, and many other organic compounds that are not waste products are usually so high as to prevent significant excretion. Accordingly, their plasma concentrations are virtually independent of renal function; i.e., the kidneys do not participate in the setting of their plasma concentrations.

Q-23 A month after 80 percent of the nephrons are destroyed, what will the blood urea concentration be, assuming it was 5 mmol/L before the disease occurred?

a 25 mmol/L
b 5 mmol/L
c 6 mmol/L
d Continuously rising
e Not calculable unless it is assumed that the patient's protein intake did not change as a result of the disease

A-23 e. If one assumes constant protein intake, 25 mmol/L would have been the correct answer since total filtered urea could be restored to normal at this point [25(0.2 × 180) = 5 × 180]. However, had protein intake been reduced by 50 percent, plasma urea would stabilize at 12.5 mmol/L since only 50 percent as much urea would be produced.

Q-24 The concentration of urea in urine is always much higher than the concentration in plasma. Is this because the overall tubular handling of urea is secretion?

A-24 No. The overall tubular handling of urea is reabsorption; i.e., reabsorption is far more extensive in the proximal tubule and collecting ducts than secretion is in the straight proximal tubule and thin loops of Henle. The reason urinary urea concentration is higher than that of plasma is that relatively more water has been reabsorbed than urea, thereby concentrating the urea in the tubule.

Q-25 If the concentration of protein in the glomerular filtrate was 0.005 g/100 mL and none was reabsorbed, how much protein would be excreted per day (assuming a normal GFR)?

A-25 9g.

$$Excreted = filtered - reabsorbed$$
$$= (0.05 \text{ g/L} \times 180 \text{ L/day}) - 0$$
$$= 9 \text{ g/day}$$

Q-26 A drug has been found to increase uric acid excretion. Give at least three ways it might act.

A-26 1. Increase uric acid synthesis → increased plasma uric acid → increased filtration
2. Stimulation of secretion
3. Inhibition of reabsorption

Q-27 If you wished to increase your patient's excretion of quinine, a weak organic base, what change in urinary pH would you try to induce?

A-27 Decreased pH. This would convert more of the quinine to its charged form and prevent its passive reabsorption.

Q-28 During a dog experiment, a clamp around the renal artery is partially tightened to reduce renal arterial pressure from a mean of 120 mmHg to 80 mmHg. How much do you predict RBF will change?

      a 33 percent decrease
      b Zero
      c 5 to 10 percent decrease
      d 33 percent increase

A-28 c. Autoregulation prevents the RBF from decreasing in direct proportion to mean arterial pressure, but autoregulation is not 100 percent.

Q-29 A patient suffers a hemorrhage that drops the mean arterial pressure by 25 percent. What do you predict happens to the GFR and RBF?
      a Almost no change
      b A fairly large decrease, RBF > GFR

A-29 b. If you answered a, you probably assumed that autoregulation would prevent any significant change. This is wrong because the drop in pressure reflexly stimulates increased sympathetic tone to the kidney (and increased plasma angiotensin II). (See text for the reason the GFR change is less than the RBF change.)

Q-30 A normal dog is given a drug that inhibits sodium chloride reabsorption by the proximal tubule. GFR decreases within seconds to a particular value and then slowly decreases even more over the next 2 h. Why?

A-30 The immediate decrease in GFR is due to tubuloglomerular feedback; the more delayed additional decrease is due to reflexly increased sympathetic outflow to the kidney, triggered by the progressive diuretic-induced depletion of bodily sodium and water.

Q-31 In the situation described in Q-29, what would happen to RBF (relative to its value following the hemorrhage) if the hemorrhaged person were given a drug that blocks synthesis of prostaglandins?
      a Increase
      b Remain the same
      c Decrease

A-31 c. Increased sympathetic outflow and increased angiotensin II induce the synthesis of vasodilator prostaglandins; the drug would prevent this and, hence, eliminate the usual prostaglandin-dependent opposition to renal vasoconstriction.

Q-32 A dog is subjected to a mild hemorrhage; its mean arterial pressure decreases slightly, and its plasma renin concentration increases markedly. It is then given a drug that blocks beta-adrenergic receptors. Its plasma renin decreases back toward the normal (prehemorrhage) values but still remains elevated to some extent. Why?

A-32 Most of the stimulus for increased renin release in this situation occurred through the renal sympathetic nerves and epinephrine, which act directly on the granular cells via beta-adrenergic receptors. Some stimulus still remains, however, via the intrarenal baroreceptors and macula densa.

Q-33 A normal person is given a drug that blocks angiotensin-converting enzyme. What happens to renin secretion?

A-33 It increases. Angiotensin II exerts a potent inhibitory effect on renin secretion; therefore, eliminating angiotensin II relieves this inhibition, resulting in more renin secretion.

Q-34 In the steady state, what is the amount of sodium chloride excreted daily in the urine by a normal person ingesting 12 g of sodium chloride per day?
a 12 g/day
b Less than 12 g/day

A-34 b. Urinary excretion in the steady state must be less than ingested sodium chloride by an amount equal to that lost in the sweat and feces. This is normally quite small, less than 1 g/day, so that urine execretion in this case equals approximately 11 g/day.

Q-35 A person's plasma sodium concentration is 144 mmol/L; inulin clearance, 120 mL/min; urine volume, 36 mL in 30 min; and urine sodium concentration, 200 mmol/L. What percentage of filtered sodium is excreted?

A-35 1.4 percent.

$$\text{Filtered Na}^+ = 144 \text{ mmol/L} \times 0.12 \text{ L/min}$$
$$= 17.28 \text{ mmol/min}$$
$$\text{Excreted Na}^+ = 0.036 \text{ L/30 min} \times 200 \text{ mmol/L}$$
$$= 0.24 \text{ mmol/min}$$
$$\% \frac{\text{excreted}}{\text{filtered}} = \frac{0.24}{17.28} \times 100 = 1.4\%$$

Q-36 In chronic renal disease, plasma urea may become markedly elevated. Under such circumstances urea will act as an osmotic diuretic. What does this do to sodium, chloride, and water excretion?

A-36 Sodium, chloride, and water excretion will all increase.

Q-37 Normally there are no *passive* fluxes of sodium into or out of the proximal tubule. True or false?

A-37 False. There are very large passive fluxes in both directions. However, there is little *net* passive flux because of the absence of a significant electrochemical gradient for sodium.

Q-38 **a** Complete inhibition of active sodium and chloride transport by the ascending loop of Henle would virtually eliminate the ability to excrete a concentrated urine. True or false?
b Increasing the passive permeability of the ascending loop to sodium and chloride would reduce the maximal concentrating ability of the kidney. True or false?
c Active reabsorption of sodium and chloride by the descending loop is a component of the countercurrent multiplier system. True or false?

A-38 a. True.
b. True. The gradient between ascending loop and interstitium at any *horizontal level* would be decreased; therefore the gradient from top to bottom would be decreased.
c. False. There is no reabsorption of sodium or chloride by the descending loop.

Q-39 A normal experimental animal is given a drug, and a sample of tubular fluid (TF) is later collected by micropuncture from the end of the proximal convoluted tubule along with a plasma (P) sample. The TF/P ratio for inulin is 1.5, and for sodium, 0.99. Has the drug inhibited, stimulated, or done nothing to proximal sodium reabsorption?

A-39 Inhibited it. The inulin data reveal that only 30 percent of filtered water has been reabsorbed. Since TF/P for sodium is essentially unity (the normal value for proximal fluid), this means that only 30 percent of the filtered sodium was reabsorbed, a value far below normal. If you are having trouble understanding this relatively difficult question, look at footnote 4 in Chap. 3.

Q-40 True or false:
   a Net reabsorption of sodium occurs in the ascending loop of Henle.
   b Net reabsorption of water occurs in the descending loop.
   c Net reabsorption of water occurs in the collecting ducts.
   d Net bulk flow of interstitial fluid into the vasa recta occurs.

A-40 All are true. The last may have given you trouble. The fact is that the vasa recta act as countercurrent exchangers to eliminate net overall *diffusion* of sodium and water into or out of the vasa recta by balancing any net movements in the descending vessels with opposite ones in the ascending. Thus, net diffusional movements are minimal, but normal capillary *bulk-flow* must still be occurring, or otherwise the sodium and water reabsorbed from the loops of Henle and collecting ducts would not be carried away.

Q-41 A drug is given that blocks sodium channels or carriers in the luminal membrane all along the nephron but does not act on the Na,K-ATPase pumps in the basolateral membrane. What happens to sodium reabsorption?

A-41 It markedly decreases or ceases completely. Even though the active step is not altered by the drug, there will be little or no sodium entering the cell to be acted on by the pumps.

Q-42 A drug is given that blocks all Na,K-ATPase sites in the nephron. Would this eliminate chloride reabsorption in all nephron segments?

A-42 Chloride reabsorption would be blocked everywhere except the cortical collecting duct. The active process for chloride in this latter segment is by countertransport with bicarbonate.

Q-43 A patient taking large quantities of aspirin for arthritis manifests an unusually persistent degree of water retention. Why might this be?

A-43 Aspirin inhibits prostaglandin synthesis; therefore, the person is hyper-responsive to ADH since ADH's partial inhibition of its own action, via stimulation of prostaglandin synthesis, is lost.

Q-44 In an experiment a dog's rate of glomerular filtration of sodium in an isolated pump-perfused kidney is found to be 15 mmol/min.
   a How much sodium do you predict remains in the tubule at the end of the proximal tubule?

b Its GFR is suddenly increased by 33 percent. How much sodium now is left at the end of the proximal tubule?

A-44 a. 5 mmol/min. Approximately two-thirds of filtered sodium is reabsorbed by the proximal tubule.

b. 6.6 mmol/min. Filtered sodium rises from 15 to 20 mmol/min. Glomerulotubular balance maintains fractional sodium reabsorption at approximately two-thirds of the filtered load.

Q-45 Normally aldosterone controls the reabsorption of approximately 33 g of sodium chloride per day. If a patient loses 100 percent of adrenal function, will 33 g of sodium chloride be excreted per day indefinitely?

A-45 No. As soon as the person starts to become sodium-deficient as a result of the increased sodium excretion, the usual sodium-retaining reflexes will be set into motion. They will, of course, be unable to raise aldosterone secretion, but they will lower GFR and alter the other factors that influence tubular sodium reabsorption to at least partially compensate for the decreased aldosterone-dependent sodium reabsorption.

Q-46 What happens to sodium excretion during quiet standing?

A-46 It decreases. Because of venous pooling of blood and increased filtration of fluid across the leg capillaries, quiet standing causes an effective decrease in plasma volume, which triggers all the described inputs leading to decreased sodium excretion (decreased GFR and increased tubular reabsorption).

Q-47 A patient has just suffered a severe hemorrhage and the plasma protein concentration is normal. (Not enough time has elapsed for interstitial fluid to move into the plasma.) Does this mean that the peritubular-capillary oncotic pressure is also normal?

A-47 No. It will probably be above normal because of increased filtration fraction secondary to sympathetically mediated renal arteriolar constriction.

Q-48 If the right renal artery becomes abnormally constricted, what will happen to renin secretion by it and by the left kidney?

A-48 The right kidney will have increased secretion because of decreased renal perfusion acting via the intrarenal baroceptor and decreased flow to the macula densa. This increased secretion will result in elevated systemic arterial angiotensin II and arterial blood pressure, both of which will inhibit renin secretion from the left kidney.

Q-49 A patient with leaky glomeruli but normal tubules loses protein in the urine and, therefore, has a plasma albumin of 2.5 g/100mL. Virtually all sodium ingested is retained (i.e., urinary excretion of sodium is close to zero) and the patient is becoming edematous. What is the stimulus for renal sodium retention in this case since total extracellular volume is clearly greater than normal?

A-49 Because of the low plasma albumin, *plasma volume* is decreased as a result of the abnormal balance of forces across capillaries. This decreased plasma volume initiates sodium-retaining reflexes just as if the plasma volume had been decreased by diarrhea, a burn, etc. The retained fluid does not restore the plasma volume to normal, however, but merely filters into the interstitium, where it increases the edema. Interestingly, tubular sodium reabsorption is increased in this state despite the fact that peritubular-capillary protein concentration is almost certainly lower than normal, which should reduce tubular sodium reabsorption. A reflexly increased aldosterone level is certainly important in stimulating sodium reabsorption and overriding this effect of the low protein. Changes in renal hemodynamics may also be important.

Q-50 A patient is suffering from primary hyperaldosteronism, i.e., increased secretion of aldosterone, usually caused by an aldosterone-producing adrenal tumor. Is plasma renin concentration higher or lower than normal?

A-50 Lower. The increased aldosterone causes positive sodium balance, which reflexly inhibits renin secretion. Thus, one observes high plasma aldosterone and low plasma renin—a strong tip-off to the presence of the disease since in almost all other situations renin and aldosterone change in the same direction (because the renin-angiotensin system is the major control of aldosterone secretion).

Q-51 Any agent that increases sodium and water excretion is called a *diuretic* (even though *natriuretic* is probably a better term). List possible mechanisms of the actions of these drugs.

A-51 1. They increase GFR either by raising blood pressure or by dilating renal afferent arterioles.
2. The above hemodynamic changes would also inhibit sodium reabsorption by increasing peritubular-capillary hydraulic pressure and/or reducing peritubular-capillary oncotic pressure (because of decreased filtration fraction).
3. They directly inhibit the active-transport system for sodium, e.g., by blocking Na,K-ATPase.
4. They directly block the Na,K,2Cl cotransporter in the thick ascending limb of Henle.
5. They directly block the Na,Cl cotransporter in the distal convoluted tubule.
6. They inhibit sodium-hydrogen-ion countertransport
7. They inhibit the H-ATPase in the collecting-duct system. (You will not know this now, but you will by the end of the book.)
8. They inhibit secretion of renin, the formation of angiotensin II, or the action of angiotensin II on the adrenal cortex.
9. They block the action of aldosterone.
10. They act as an osmotic diuretic by their osmotic contribution (mannitol, for example).
   This list is by no means exhaustive but does include the major clinically useful types of diuretics.

Q-52 A normal subject loses 2 L of isotonic salt solution because of diarrhea. He or she simultaneously drinks 2 L of pure water. What happens to
a Extracellular fluid volume

b Body fluid osmolarity
c Renin and aldosterone secretion
d ADH secretion

A-52 a and b. Extracellular volume and osmolarity both decrease. The entire 2 L of solution was lost from the extracellular compartment since it was isotonic. (Therefore, osmolarity did not change, and no water moved into or out of cells.) The 2 L of ingested pure water is distributed throughout the bodily water, only about one-third remaining in the extracellular fluid. Moreover, the addition of pure water lowers the osmolarity.

c. This increases because of reflexes induced by the decreased extracellular volume.

d. We cannot predict for certain, but it probably decreases. The decreased extracellular volume reflexly stimulates ADH secretion, but the reduced osmolarity should inhibit it via the hypothalamic osmoreceptors. The osmoreceptor input usually predominates during such "conflicts" unless the extracellular volume depletion is very large.

Q-53 A person excretes 2 L of urine having an osmolarity of 600 mosmol/L. As a result, does bodily fluid osmolarity *increase* or *decrease*?

A-53 Decrease. He or she has excreted 2 L × 600 mosmol/L = 1200 mosmol total solute and 2 L water. Two liters of normal bodily fluids contain 2 L × 300 mosmol/L = 600 mosmol solutes. Accordingly, he or she has excreted relatively more solute than water, compared to the normal proportions in the bodily fluids. This will reduce the bodily fluid osmolarity.

Q-54 A person excretes 3 L of urine having an osmolarity of 150 mosmol/L. As a result, does bodily fluid osmolarity *increase* or *decrease*?

A-54 Increase. He or she has excreted 3 L × 150 mosmol/L = 450 mosmol total solute, and 3 L water have been excreted. This amount of solute is contained in 450 mosmol ÷ 300 mosmol/L = 1.5 L normal body fluid. Therefore he or she has excreted relatively more water than solute, compared to the normal proportions in the bodily fluids.

Q-55 What are the major renal sites of action of the following hormones?
Aldosterone
ADH
Renin
Epinephrine
Angiotensin II

A-55 Aldosterone: Cortical collecting duct
ADH: Cortical and medullary collecting ducts
Renin: No renal site of action
Epinephrine: Renal arterioles, JG apparatus, and renal tubules (mainly proximal tubule)
Angiotensin II: Renal arterioles and renal tubules (mainly proximal tubule)

Q-56 What are the major controls of aldosterone secretion?

A-56 1. Angiotensin II
         2. ACTH
         3. Plasma sodium concentration
         4. Plasma potassium concentration

Q-57 What are the major controls of renin secretion?
A-57 1. Afferent-arteriolar pressure (intrarenal baroreceptor)
         2. Sodium chloride load to the macula densa
         3. Activity of renal sympathetic nerves
         4. Angiotensin II

Q-58 What are the major controls of ADH secretion?
A-58 1. Bodily fluid osmolarity via hypothalamic osmoreceptors
         2. Plasma volume (via cardiovascular baroreceptors)

Q-59 Control of potassium excretion is achieved mainly by regulating the rate of
        a Potassium filtration
        b Potassium reabsorption
        c Potassium secretion
A-59 c.

Q-60 A person in previously normal potassium balance maintains neurotic hyperventilation for several days. During this period what happens to potassium balance?
A-60 It becomes negative. The hyperventilation causes alkalosis, which in turn induces increased secretion of potassium (probably because of an alkalosis-induced elevation of renal-tubular cell potassium concentration).

Q-61 A patient has a tumor in the adrenal that continuously secretes large quantities of aldosterone (primary hyperaldosteronism). Is the rate of potassium excretion normal, high, or low?
A-61 High. The increased aldosterone stimulates potassium secretion and, thereby, excretion. Moreover, once enough sodium has been retained to increase GFR and to cause partial inhibition of proximal and loop sodium reabsorption, the increased delivery of fluid to the cortical collecting duct further enhances potassium secretion. There is no potassium escape similar to the sodium escape from aldosterone.

Q-62 A patient with severe congestive heart failure is secreting large quantities of aldosterone. Is the rate of potassium excretion normal, high, or low?
A-62 Relatively normal. You may well have answered "high", assuming that the increased aldosterone would stimulate potassium secretion, as in the previous question. However, this effect is more than balanced by the fact that the patient has a decrease in both GFR and flow of fluid into the cortical collecting duct (because of increased proximal and loop reabsorption); recall that potassium secretion is impaired when the amount of fluid flowing through the cortical collecting duct is reduced. This explains why patients with the diseases of secondary hyperaldosteronism with edema do

not lose large quantities of potassium, whereas patients with primary hyperaldosteronism do.

Q-63 Give three reasons why osmotic diuresis (as, for example, in uncontrolled diabetic ketoacidosis) enhances potassium excretion.

A-63
1. It inhibits potassium reabsorption by the proximal tubule.
2. It increases fluid delivery to the cortical collecting duct, resulting in increased potassium secretion.
3. It causes sodium depletion, which increases aldosterone secretion (via the renin-angiotensin system), and this hormone stimulates potassium secretion.

Q-64 A patient is observed to excrete 2 L of alkaline (pH = 7.6) urine having a bicarbonate concentration of 28 mmol/L. The rate of titratable-acid excretion is

a 56 mmol
b Negative
c Cannot tell without data for ammonium

A-64 b. If the urine has a pH greater than 7.4, clearly there is no titratable acid (t.a.) excreted; indeed, there is negative t.a. excretion. Ammonium does not contribute to t.a. and may be ignored in the calculation of t.a.

Q-65 The following data are obtained for a subject:

$$C_{In} = 170 \text{ L/day}$$
$$P_{HCO_3^-} = 25 \text{ mmol/L}$$
$$U_{HCO_3^-} = 0$$
$$\text{Urine pH} = 5.8$$
$$\text{Titratable acid} = 26 \text{ mmol/day}$$
$$\text{Urine NH}_4^+ = 48 \text{ mmol/day}$$

Calculate the amount of new bicarbonate added to the blood, i.e., acid excreted.

A-65 74 mmol/day (sum of t.a. and NH_4^+, minus bicarbonate excreted).

Q-66 Which values could you predict are those for a patient with primary hyperaldosteronism?

	Urine pH	Plasma pH
a	6.9	7.55
b	8.2	7.55
c	4.8	7.30

A-66 a. This patient secretes excessive amounts of aldosterone, which induces potassium deficiency (because of increased renal potassium secretion). The potassium deficiency and aldosterone together then induce inappropriately large renal hydrogen-ion secretion, thereby producing a metabolic alkalosis. Note that the urine is still acid; i.e., the kidneys are not compensating for the alkalosis.

Q-67 What are the three direct effects of aldosterone on the tubule?

A-67 Increased sodium reabsorption, increased potassium secretion, and increased hydrogen-ion secretion.

Q-68 A patient has been losing large amounts of HCl because of persistent vomiting for 3 days and, therefore, has a plasma pH of 7.50. The urine pH was 8.0 at the end of day 1 and 6.9 at the end of day 3. Explain.

A-68 The alkaline urine on day 1 is the appropriate renal compensation for vomiting-induced alkalosis. The slightly acid urine on day 3 signifies that the kidneys are no longer compensating for alkalosis. This happens mainly because the progressive development of severe extracellular volume contraction and chloride depletion stimulates proximal hydrogen-ion secretion, preventing loss of bicarbonate in the urine. (Potassium depletion and increased aldosterone may also contribute.)

Q-69 Match the top (lettered) column with the bottom (numbered) column ("increased" or "decreased" is used with reference to normal).
  a Diabetic ketoacidosis
  b Hypoventilation
  c Excessive ingestion of sodium bicarbonate
  1 Increased plasma pH, increased plasma bicarbonate, alkaline urine
  2 Decreased plasma pH, decreased plasma bicarbonate, acidic urine
  3 Decreased plasma pH, increased plasma bicarbonate, acidic urine

A-69 a. 2
  b. 3
  c. 1

Q-70 Which of the following would you expect to find in a patient suffering from primary hypersecretion of parathyroid hormone?
  a Increased plasma calcium
  b Decreased plasma phosphate
  c Increased urine calcium
  d Increased tubular reabsorption of calcium
  e Increased urine phosphate
  f Increased plasma calcitonin
  g Increased plasma $1,25\text{-}(OH)_2D_3$

A-70 All are correct; c and d are not mutually exclusive because of the marked increase in filtered calcium. Calcitonin is reflexly increased by the increased plasma calcium. Formation of $1,25\text{-}(OH)_2D_3$ is enhanced by parathyroid hormone.

Q-71 Which of the following would you expect to find in a person whose kidneys could not synthesize $1,25\text{-}(OH)_2D_3$?
  a Decreased gastointestinal absorption of calcium
  b Decreased gastointestinal absorption of phosphate
  c Decreased plasma calcium concentration
  d Increased plasma parathyroid-hormone concentration

A-71 All. The increased parathyroid-hormone secretion is stimulated by the low plasma calcium.

Q-72 Complete inhibition of active sodium reabsorption would cause an increase in the excretion of which of the following substances?

a   Water
b   Urea
c   Chloride
d   Glucose
e   Amino acids
f   Potassium
g   Bicarbonate
h   Calcium

A-72 All. The reasons are all given in relevant sections of the text.

Appendix A

CLASSES OF DIURETICS

Class	Mechanism	Major site affected
Carbonic anhydrase inhibitors	Inhibit secretion of hydrogen ions, which causes less reabsorption of bicarbonate and sodium	Proximal tubule
Loop diuretics	Inhibit Na, K, 2Cl cotransporter in luminal membrane	Thick ascending loop of Henle
Thiazides	Inhibit Na, Cl cotransporter in luminal membrane	Distal convoluted tubule
Potassium-sparing diuretics*	Inhibit action of aldosterone	Cortical collecting duct
	Block sodium channels in luminal membrane	Collecting-duct system

*Except for this category, diuretics increase potassium excretion as well as sodium excretion (see text for discussion of the reasons for this increase). Aldosterone antagonists do not increase potassium excretion because they inhibit aldosterone's stimulation of potassium secretion. The sodium channel blockers also inhibit potassium secretion, in this case by reducing the amount of sodium entering the cortical collecting duct cell for transport across the basolateral membrane by the Na, K-ATPase pumps; this reduces the activity of the pumps and, hence, the active transport of potassium into the cell.

Appendix B

FIGURES SUMMARIZING ELECTROLYTE TRANSPORT BY DIFFERENT TUBULAR CELL TYPES

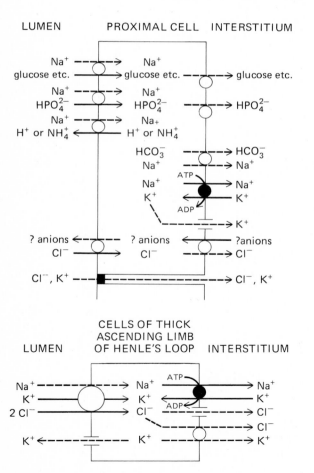

DISTAL CONVOLUTED CELL

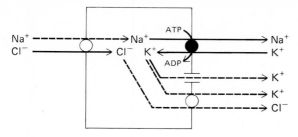

PRINCIPAL CELL OF CORTICAL COLLECTING DUCT

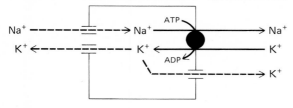

HYDROGEN-ION-SECRETING INTERCALATED CELL OF CORTICAL AND MEDULLARY COLLECTING DUCTS

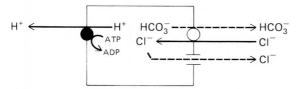

These cells can also reabsorb potassium,
and the following is an alternative model,
in which the key element is an H-K-ATPase pump.

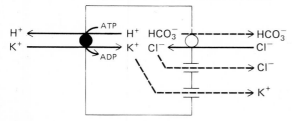

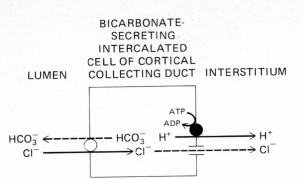

SUGGESTED READINGS

RESEARCH TECHNIQUES

Burg M: Introduction: background and development of microperfusion technique. *Kidney Int* 1982;22:417.

Fine LG (ed): Renal cells in culture. *Mineral and Electrolyte Metabolism* 1986; 12(1):5.

Palmer L: Patch-clamp technique in renal physiology. *Am J Physiol* 1986; 250:F379.

Symposium on methods in renal research. *Kidney Int* 1986;30:141

ANALYSIS OF INDIVIDUAL NEPHRON SEGMENTS

Chapters 6 to 10 concern the renal handling of specific substances. Another organizational approach to renal physiology is to look at a particular nephron segment and describe its various transport characteristics. The Suggested Readings in this section, based largely on isolated-perfused-tubule work, follow this pattern.

Berry CA: Heterogeneity of tubular transport processes in the nephron. *Ann Rev Physiol* 1982;44:181.

Jacobson HR: Functional segmentation of the mammalian nephron. *Am J Physiol* 1981;241:F205.

Koeppen BM, Biagi BA, Giebisch G: Electrophysiology of mammalian renal tubules. *Ann Rev Physiol* 1983;45:483.

Madsen KM, Tisher CC: Structural-functional relationships along the distal nephron. *Am J Physiol* 1986;250:F-1.

Transport characteristics of nephron segments (a symposium). *Kidney Int* 1982;22:425.

Walker LA, Valtin H: Biological importance of nephron heterogeneity. *Ann Rev Physiol* 1982;44:203.

211

CHAP. 1

Barajas L: Anatomy of the juxtaglomerular apparatus. *Am J Physiol* 1979; 237:F333.

Beeuwkes R III: The vascular organization of the kidney. *Ann Rev Physiol* 1980;42:531.

Bonvalet J-P, Pradelles P, Farman N: Segmental synthesis and actions of prostaglandins along the nephron. *Am J Physiol* 1987;253:F377.

Bulger RE, Dobyan DC: Recent advances in renal morphology. *Ann Rev Physiol* 1982;44:147.

Dzau VJ, Burt DW, Pratt RE: Molecular biology of the renin-angiotensin system. *Am J Physiol* 1988;255:F563.

Ganong WF: The brain renin-angiotensin system. *Ann Rev Physiol* 1984;46:17.

Kriz W, Bankir L: A standard nomenclature for structures of the kidney. *Am J Physiol* 1988;254:F1.

Makhoul RG, Gewertz BL: Renal prostaglandins. *J Surg Res* 1986;40:181.

Nasjlette A, Malik KU: The renal kallikrein-kinin and prostaglandin systems interactions. *Ann Rev Physiol* 1981;81:597.

Prostaglandins and the kidney (a symposium). *Kidney Int* 1981;19:755.

Scicli AG, Carretero OA: Renal kallikrein-kinin system. *Kidney Int* 1986;29:120.

Tisher CC: Anatomy of the kidney, in Brenner BM, Rector FC (eds): *The Kidney.* Philadelphia, Saunders, 1981.

CHAP. 2

Abrahamson DR: Structure and development of the glomerular capillary wall and basement membrane. *Am J Physiol* 1987;253:F783.

Arendshorst WJ, Gottschalk CW: Glomerular ultrafiltration dynamics: historical perspective. *Am J Physiol* 1985;248:F163.

Aronson PS: Identifying secondary active solute transport in epithelia. *Am J Physiol* 1981;240:F1.

Brenner BM, Humes HD: Mechanics of glomerular ultrafiltration. *N Engl J Med* 1977;297:148.

Deen, WM, Robertson CR, Brenner BM: Glomerular utrafiltration. *Fed Proc* 1974;33:14.

Geck P, Heinz E: Secondary active transport: introductory remarks. *Kidney Int* 1989;36:334–341.

Giebisch G, Boulpaep E (eds). Symposium on cotransport mechanisms in renal tubules. *Kidney Int* 1989;36:333.

Kreisberg JI, Venkatachalam M, Troyer D: Contractile properties of cultured glomerular mesangial cells. *Am J Physiol* 1985;249:F457.

Oken DE: An analysis of glomerular dynamics in rat, dog, and man. *Kidney Int* 1982;22:136.

Pappenheimer JR: Passage of molecules through capillary walls. *Physiol Rev* 1953;33:387.

Schafer, JA: Membrane transport, in Klahr S, Massry SG (eds): *Contemporary Nephrology.* New York, Plenum, 1981, vol 1.

CHAP. 3

Kassirer JP: Clinical evaluation of kidney function: glomerular function. *N Engl J Med* 1971;285:385.

Levinsky NG, Levy M: Clearance techniques, in Berliner RW, Orloff J (eds): *Handbook of Renal Physiology*. Washington, DC, American Physiological Society, 1973, sec 8.

Maack T: Renal clearance and isolated kidney perfusion techniques. *Kidney Int* 1986;30:142.

Smith HW: *Principles of Renal Physiology*. New York, Oxford, 1956, chaps 3–6.

CHAP. 4

Biber J: Cellular aspects of proximal tubular phosphate reabsorption. *Kidney Int* 1989;36:360.

Ganapathy V, Leibach FH: Carrier-mediated reabsorption of small peptides in renal proximal tubule. *Am J Physiol* 1986;251:F945.

Gregor R, Lang F, Silbernagls: *Renal Transport of Organic Substances*. New York, Springer-Verlag, 1981.

Guggino WB, Guggino SE: Renal anion transport. *Kidney Int* 1989;36:385.

Kahn AM: Indirect coupling between sodium and urate transport in the proximal tubule. *Kidney Int* 1989;36:378.

Knepper MA, Roch-Ramel F: Pathways of urea transport in the mammalian kidney. *Kidney Int* 1987;31:629.

Moller JV, Sheikh MI: Renal organic anion transport system: pharmacological, physiological, and biochemical aspects. *Pharm Rev* 1983;34:315.

Rabkin R, Glaser T, Petersen J: Renal peptide hormone metabolism. *The Kidney* 1983;16:25–29.

Saktor B: Sodium-coupled hexose transport. *Kidney Int* 1989;36:342.

Schafer JA, Barfuss DW: Membrane mechanisms for transepithelial amino acid absorption and secretion. *Am J Physiol* 1980;238:F335.

Schafer JA, Williams JC Jr: Transport of metabolic substrates by the proximal nephron. *Ann Rev Physiol* 1985;47:103.

Silbernagl S: Tubular reabsorption of amino acids in the kidney. *NIPS* 1986;1:167–172.

Zelikovic I, Chesney RW: Sodium-coupled amino acid transport in renal tubule. *Kidney Int* 1989;36:351.

CHAP. 5

Baylis C, Blantz RC: Glomerular hemodynamics. *NIPS* 1986;1:86–89.

Blantz RC, Pelayo JC: A functional role for the tubuloglomerular feedback mechanism *Kidney Int* 1984;25:739.

Bonvalet J-P, Pradelles P, Farman N: Segmental synthesis and actions of prostaglandins along the nephron. *Am J Physiol* 1987;253:F377.

Brenner BM (ed): Control of glomerular function by intrinsic contractile elements (a symposium). *Fed Proc* 1983;42:3045.

Briggs JP, Schnermann J: Macula densa control of renin secretion and glomerular vascular tone: evidence for common cellular mechanisms. *Renal Physiol* 1986;9:193.

Briggs JP, Schnermann J: The tubuloglomerular feedback mechanism: functional and biochemical aspects. *Ann Rev Physiol* 1986;49:251.

Churchill PC: Second messengers in renin secretion. *Am J Physiol* 1985;249:F175.

Dworkin LD, Ilkuni I, Brenner BM: Hormonal modulation of glomerular function. *Am J Physiol* 1983;244:F95.

Henrich WL: Role of prostaglandins in renin secretion. *Kidney Int* 1981;19:822.

Hsueh WA: Potential effects of renin activation on the regulation of renin production. *Am J Physiol* 1984;247:F205.

Keeton TK, Campbell WB: Control of renin release and its alteration by drugs, *Cardiovascular Pharmacology*. New York, Raven Press, 1984, 2d ed, pp 65–118.

Lee MR: Dopamine and the kidney. *Clin Sci* 1982;62:439.

Loutzenhiser R, Epstein M: Effects of calcium antagonists on renal hemodynamics. *Am J Physiol* 1985;249:F619.

Navar LG: Physiological role of the intrarenal renin-angiotensin system (a symposium). *Fed Proc* 1986;45:1411.

Schlondorff D: The golmerular mesangial cell: an expanding role for a specialized pericyte. *FASEB J* 1987;1:272.

Schnermann J, Briggs J: Function of the juxtaglomerular apparatus: local control of glomerular hemodynamics. *The Kidney* 1985;28:669.

Scicli AG, Carretero OA: Renal kallikrein-kinin system. *Kidney Int* 1986;29:120.

Skott O: Do osmotic forces play a role in renin secretion? *Am J Physiol* 1988;255:F1.

Spielman WS, Thompson CI: A proposed role for adenosine in the regulation of renal hemodynamics and renin release. *Am J Physiol* 1982;242:F243.

CHAP. 6

Abramov M, Beauvens R, Cogan E: Cellular events in vasopressin action. *Kidney Int* 1987;32(suppl 21): J-56.

Berry CA, Rector FC Jr: Electroneutral NaCl absorption in the proximal tubule: mechanisms of apical Na-coupled transport. *Kidney Int* 1988;36:403.

Culpepper RM: Na^+-K^+-2 Cl^- cotransport in the thick ascending limb of Henle. *Hospital Practice* 1989 (June 15); 217–242.

deRouffignac C, Jamison RL: Symposium on the urinary concentrating mechanism. *Kidney Int* 1987;31:501.

Dubinsky WP Jr: The physiology of epithelial chloride channels. *Hospital Practice* 1989 (Jan. 15); 69–80.

Fromter E, Sauer F: Theoretical basis of electrophysiologic analysis of transepithelial transport, in Seldin DW, Grebisch G (eds): *The Kidney: Physiology and Pathophysiology*. New York, Raven Press, 1985, vol 1.

Greger R: Ion transport mechanisms in thick ascending limb of Henle's loop. *Physiol Rev* 1985;65:760.

Greger R: Chloride transport in thick ascending limb, distal convolution, and collecting duct. *Ann Rev Physiol* 1988;50:111.

Handler JS: Antidiuretic hormone moves membranes. *Am J Physiol* 1988; 255:F375.

Jacobson HR: Functional segmentation of the mammalian nephron. *Am J Physiol* 1981;241:F205.

Jamison RJ: The renal concentrating mechanism. *Kidney Int* 1987;32(suppl 21): S-43.

Jorgensen PL: Structure, function and regulation of Na,K-ATPase in the kidney. *Kidney Int* 1986;29:10.

Karniski LP, Aronson PS: Formate: A critical intermediate for chloride transport in the proximal tubule. *NIPS* 1987;2:160–164.

Kinter LB, Huffman WF, Stassen FL: Antagonists of the antidiuretic activity of vasopressin. *Am J Physiol* 1988;254:F165.

Knepper M, Burg M: Organization of nephron function. *Am J Physiol* 1983;244:F579.

Kokko JP: The role of the collecting duct in urinary concentration. *Kidney Int* 1987;31:606.

Kramer HJ, Glanzer K, Dusing R: Role of prostaglandins in the regulation of renal water excretion. *Kidney Int* 1981;19:851.

Lang F, Messner G, Rehwald W: Electrophysiology of sodium-coupled transport in proximal renal tubules. *Am J Physiol* 1986;250:F953.

Maddox DA, Gennari JF: The early proximal tubule: a high-capacity delivery-responsive reabsorptive site. *Am J Physiol* 1987;252:F573.

Madsen KM, Tisher CG: Structural-functional relationships along the distal nephron. *Am J Physiol* 1986;250:F1.

Molony DA, Reeves WB, Andreoli TE: $Na^+K^+:2Cl^-$ cotransport and the thick ascending limb. *Kidney Int* 1989;36:418.

O'Grady SM, Palfrey HC, Field M: Characteristics and functions of Na-K-Cl cotransport in epithelial tissues. *Am J Physiol* 1987;253:C177.

Rector FC Jr: Sodium, bicarbonate, and chloride absorption by the proximal tubule. *Am J Physiol* 1983;244:F461.

Roy DR, Jamison RL: Countercurrent system and its regulation, in Seldin DW, Giebisch G (eds): *The Kidney: Physiology and Pathophysiology*. New York, Raven Press, 1985, vol. 1.

Schafer JA: Mechanisms coupling the absorption of solutes and water in the proximal nephron. *Kidney Int* 1984;25:708.

Schafer JA: Fluid absorption in the kidney proximal tubule. *NIPS* 1987;2:22.

Schild L, Giebisch G: Chloride transport in the proximal renal tubule. *Ann Rev Physiol* 1988;50:97.

Schrier RW, Linas LS: Mechanism of the defect in water excretion in adrenal insufficiency. *Min Elect Met* 1980;4:1.

Schuster VL, Stokes JB: Chloride transport by the cortical and outer medullary collecting duct. *Am J Physiol* 1987;253:F203.

Stokes JB: Electroneutral NaCl transport in the distal tubule. *Kidney Int* 1989;36:427.

vanDriesche W, Zeiske W: Ionic channels in epithelial cell membranes. *Physiol Rev* 1985;65:833.

See also articles under Analysis of Individual Nephron Segments.

CHAP. 7

Blaine EH (ed): Atrial natriuretic factor (a symposium). *Fed Proc* 1986;45:2360.

Blessing WW: Central neurotransmitter pathways for baroreceptor-initiated secretion of vasopressin. *NIPS* 1986;1:90–91.

Bonvalet J-P, Pradelles P, Farman N: Sigmental synthesis and actions of prostaglandins along the nephron. *Am J Physiol* 1987;253:F377–387.

Carey RM, Sen S: Recent progress in the control of aldosterone secretion. *Rec Prog Horm Res* 1986;42:251.

Cowley AW Jr, Quillen EW Jr, Skelton MM: Role of vasopressin in cardiovascular regulation. *Fed Proc* 1983;42:3170.

deRouffignac C, Elalouf J-M: Hormonal regulation of chloride transport in the proximal and distal nephron. *Ann Rev Physiol* 1988;50:123.

Dewardener HE, Clarkson EM: Concept of natriuretic hormone. *Physiol Rev* 1985;65:658.

Dibona GF: Neural regulation of renal tubular sodium reabsorption and renin secretion. *Fed Proc* 1985;44:2816.

Dibona GF: Neural mechanisms in body fluid homeostasis. *Fed Proc* 1986;45:2871.

Doucet A: Multiple hormonal control of kidney tubular functions. *Am Physiol Soc* 1987;2:141.

Douglas JG: Regulation of angiotensin receptors. *NIPS* 1986;1:67.

Dzau VJ: Renal and circulatory mechanisms in congestive heart failure. *Kidney Int* 1987;31:1402.

Fitzsimons JT: Physiology and pathology of thirst and sodium appetite, in Seldin DW, Gilbisch G (eds): *The Kidney: Physiology and Pathophysiology*. New York, Raven Press, 1985, vol 1.

Fregly MJ, Rowland NE: Hormonal and neural mechanisms of sodium appetite. *NIPS* 1986;1:51–54.

Garty H, Benos DJ: Characteristics and regulatory mechanisms of the amiloride-blockable Na^+ channel. *Physiol Rev* 1988;68:309.

Genest J, Cantin M: Regulation of body fluid volume: the atrial natriuretic factor. *NIPS* 1986;1:3–5.

Goetz KL: Physiology and pathophysiology of atrial peptide. *Am J Physiol* 1988;254:E1.

Gonzalez-Campoy JM, Romero JC, Knox FG: Escape from the sodium-retaining effects of mineralcorticoids: role of ANF and intrarenal hormone systems. *Kidney Int* 1986;35:767.

Granger JP: Regulation of sodium excretion by renal interstitial hydrostatic pressure. *Fed Proc* 1986;45:2892.

Graves JW, Williams GH: Endogenous digitalis-like natriuretic factors. *Ann Rev Med* 1987;38:433.

Hall JE: Control of sodium excretion by angiotensin II: intrarenal mechanisms and blood pressure regulation. *Am J Physiol* 1986;250:R960.

Hamlyn JM, Blaustein MP: Sodium chloride, extracellular fluid volume, and blood pressure regulation. *Am J Physiol* 1986;251:F563.

Harris PJ, Navar LG: Tubular transport responses to angiotensin. *Am J Physiol* 1985;248:F621.

Hebert SC, Andreoli TE: Control of NaCl transport in the thick ascending limb. *Am J Physiol* 1984;246:F745.

Knox FG, Granger JP: Control of sodium excretion: the kidney produces under pressure. *NIPS* 1988;2:26.

Koepke JP, Dibona GF: Functions of the renal nerves. *The Physiologist* 1985;28:47.

Ledenghem JGG (ed): Symposium on Angiotensin, ACE inhibition, and the kidney. *Kidney Int* 1987;31(suppl 20):S-1.

Ledsome JR: Atrial receptors, vasopressin and blood volume in the dog. *Life Sciences* 1985;36:1315.

Maack T, et al.: Atrial natriuretic factor: Structure and functional properties. *Kidney Int* 1985;27:607.

McDougall JG: The physiology of aldosterone secretion. *NIPS* 1987;2:126.

Madsen KM, Tisher CG: Structural-functional relationships along the distal nephron. *Am J Physiol* 1986;250:F1.

Mann JFE, Johnson AK, Ganten D, Ritz E: Thirst and the renin-angiotensin system. *Kidney Int* 1987;32(suppl 21):S-27.

Menninger RP: Current concepts of volume receptor regulation of vasopressin release. *Fed Proc.* 1985;44:55.

Morel F, Doucet A: Hormonal control of kidney functions at the cell level. *Physiol Rev.* 1986;66:377.

Quinn SJ: Regulation of aldosterone secretion. *Ann Rev Physiol* 1988;50:409.

Raymond KH, Lifschitz MD: Effect of prostaglandins on renal salt and water excretion *Am J Med.* 1986;86(suppl A):22.

Reid IA: Actions of angiotensin II on the brain: mechanisms and physiologic role. *Am J Physiol* 1984;246:F533.

Robertson GL: Physiology of ADH secretion. *Kidney Int* 1988;32(suppl 21):S-20.

Roman RJ: Pressure diuresis mechanism in the control of renal function and arterial pressure. *Fed Proc.* 1986;45:2878.

Sawchenko PE, Friedman MI: Sensory functions of the liver—a review. *Am J Physiol* 1979;236:R5.

Seldin DW, Giebisch G: *The Regulation of Sodium and Chloride Balance.* New York, Raven Press, 1989.

Stanton BA: Role of adrenal hormones in regulating distal nephron structure and ion transport. *Fed Proc* 1985;44:2717.

Weingartner H, et al.: Effects of vasopressin on human memory functions. *Science* 1981;211:601.

CHAP. 8

Adrogue HJ, Madias NE: Changes in plasma potassium concentration during acute acid-base disturbances. *Am J Med* 1981;71:456.

Epstein FH, Rosa RM: Adrenergic control of serum potassium. *N Eng J Med* 1983;309:1450–1451.

Field MJ, Giebisch G: Hormonal control of renal potassium excretion. *Kidney Int* 1985;27:379.

Gennari FJ, Cohen JJ: Role of the kidney in potassium homeostasis: lessons from acid-base disturbances. *Kidney Int* 1975;8:1.

Greger R, Gogelein R: Role of K$^+$ conductive pathways in the nephron. *Kidney Int* 1987;31:1055.

Hayslett JP, Binder HJ: Mechanism of potassium adaptation. *Am J Physiol* 1982;243:F103.

Hunter M, Kawahara K, Giebisch G: Potassium channels along the nephron. *Fed Proc 1986;45:2723.*

Jacobson HR: Functional segmentation of the mammalian nephron. *Am J Physiol* 1981;241:F205.

Jamison RL: Potassium recycling. *Kidney Int* 1987;31:695.

Jamison RL, Work J, Schafer JA: New pathways for potassium transport in the kidney. *Am J Physiol* 1982;242:F297.

Madsen KM, Tisher CG: Structural-functional relationships along the distal nephron. *Am J Physiol* 1986;250:F1.

Seldin DW (ed): *The Regulation of Potassium Balance.* New York, Raven Press, 1988.

Stearns RH, et al: Internal potassium balance and the control of the plasma potassium concentration. *Medicine* 1981;60:339.

Thier SO: Potassium physiology. *Am J Med* 1986;80(suppl 4A):3.

Warnock DG, Eveloff J: K-Cl cotransport systems. *Kidney Int* 1989;36:412.

Wright FS, Giebisch G: Renal potassium transport: contributions of different nephron segments and populations. *Am J Physiol* 1978;235:F515.

Young DB: Analysis of long-term potassium regulation. *Endocrine Reviews* 1985;6:24.

Young DB: Quantitative analysis of aldosterone's role in potassium regulation. *Am J Physiol* 1988;255:F811.

See also articles listed under Analysis of Individual Nephron Segments.

CHAP. 9

Al-Awqati Q: The cellular renal response to respiratory acid-base disorders. *Kidney Int* 1985;28:845.

Aronson PS: Mechanisms of active H$^+$ secretion in the proximal tubule. *Am J Physiol* 1983;245:F647.

Arruda JAL, Kurtzman NA: Relationship of renal sodium and water transport to hydrogen ion secretion. *Ann Rev Physiol* 1978;40:43.

Arruda JAL, Kurtzman NA: Mechanisms and classification of deranged distal urinary acidification. *Am J Physiol* 1980;239:F515.

Atkinson DE, Bourke E: Metabolic aspects of the regulation of systemic pH. *Am J Physiol* 1987;252:F947.

Boron WF, Boulpaep EL: The electrogenic Na/HCO$_3$ cotransporter. *Kidney Int* 1989;36:392.

Cogan MG, Alpern RJ: Regulation of proximal bicarbonate reabsorption. *Am J Physiol* 1984;247:F387.

Dobyan DC, Bulger RE: Renal carbonic anhydrase. *Am J Physiol* 1982;243:F311.

DuBose TD Jr: Kinetics of CO_2 exchange in the kidney. *Ann Rev Phys* 1988;50:653.

Galla JH, Luke RG: Pathophysiology of metabolic alkalosis. *Hospital Practice* 1987 (Oct. 15):123–145.

Galla JH, Luke RG: Chloride transport and disorders of acid-base balance. *Ann Rev Phys* 1989;50:141.

Gennari FJ, Maddox DA, Atherton LJ, Deen WM: High P_{CO_2} in rat kidney. *NIPS* 1986;1:137–139.

Gluck SL: Cellular and molecular aspects of renal H^+ transport. *Hospital Practice* 1989 (May 15): 149–166.

Hamm LL, Simon EE: Roles and mechanisms of urinary buffer excretion. *Am J Physiol* 1987;253:F595.

Harrington JT: Metabolic alkalosis. *Kidney Int* 1984;26:88.

Hulter HN: Effects and interrelationships of PTH, Ca^{2+}, vitamin D, and P_i in acid-base homeostasis. *Am J Physiol* 1985;248:F739–752.

Knepper MA, Packer R, Good DW: Ammonium transport in the kidney. *Physiol Rev* 1989;69:179.

Levine DZ, Jacobson HR: The regulation of renal acid secretion: New observations from studies of distal nephron segments. *Kidney Int* 1986;29:1099.

Madias NE, Androgue HJ, Cohen JJ: Maladaptive renal response to secondary hypercapnia in chronic metabolic alkalosis. *Am J Physiol* 1980;238:F283.

Madsen KM, Tisher CG: Structural-functional relationships along the distal nephron. *Am J Physiol* 1986;250:F1.

Preisig PA, Alpern RJ: Basolateral membrane $H-OH-HCO_3$ transport in the proximal tubule. *Am J Physiol* 1989;256:F751.

Rector FC Jr: Sodium, bicarbonate, and chloride reabsorption by the proximal tubule. *Am J Physiol* 1983;244:F461.

Sabatini S, Kurtzman NA: The maintenance of metabolic alkalosis: factors which decrease bicarbonate excretion. *Kidney Int* 1984;25:357.

Seldin DW, Giebisch G (eds): *The Regulation of Acid-base Balance*. New York, Raven Press, 1988.

Steinmetz PR: Cellular organization of urinary acidification. *Am J Physiol* 1986;251:F173.

Tannen RL, Sastrasinh S: Response of ammonia metabolism to acute acidosis. *Kidney Int* 1984;25:1.

Walser M: Roles of urea production, ammonium excretion, and amino acid oxidation in acid-base balance. *Am J Physiol* 1986;250:F181.

Weinman EJ, Dubinsky WP Jr, Shenolikar S: *Hospital Practice* 1989 (March 15): 157–174.

Welbourne TC: Interorgan glutamine flow in metabolic acidosis. *Am J Physiol* 1989; 253:F1069.

See also articles listed under Analysis of Individual Nephron Segments.

CHAP. 10

Austin LA, Heath H III: Calcitonin: physiology and pathophysiology. *N Engl J Med* 1981;304:269.

Fraser DR: Regulation of the metabolism of vitamin D. *Physiol Rev* 1980;60:550.

Friedman P: Renal calcium transport sites and insights. *NIPS* 1988;3:17.

Gmaj P, Murer H: Cellular mechanisms of inorganic phosphate transport in kidney. *Physiol Rev* 1986;66:36.

Hammerman MR: Phosphate transport across renal proximal tubular cell membranes. *Am J Physiol* 1986;251:F385.

Holick MF: Vitamin D and the kidney. *Kidney Int* 1987;32:912.

Kawashima H, Kurokawa K: Metabolism and sites of action of vitamin D in the kidney. *Kidney Int* 1986;29:98.

Lang F, Greger R, Knox FG, Oberleithner H: Factors modulating the renal handling of phosphate. *Renal Physiol* 1981;4:1.

Lemann J Jr, Adams ND, Gray RW: Urinary calcium excretion in human beings. *N Engl J Med* 1979;301:535.

Mizzala CL, Quamme GA: Renal handling of phosphate. *Physiol Rev* 1985;65:431.

Muer H, Malmstrom K: How renal phosphate transport is regulated. *NIPS* 1987;2:45–48.

Ng RCK, Peraino RA, Suki WN: Divalent cation transport in isolated tubules. *Kidney Int* 1982;22:492.

Norman AW: The vitamin D endocrine system. *The Physiologist* 1985;28:219.

Quamme GA, Dirks JH: Magnesium transport in the nephron. *Am J Physiol* 1980;239:F393.

Suki WN: Calcium transport in the nephron. *Am J Physiol* 1979;237:F1.

Suki WN, Rouse D: Mechanisms of calcium transport. *Min Elect Met* 1981;5:175.

See also articles listed under Analysis of Individual Nephron Segments.

APPENDIX A

Jacobson HR: Diuretics: mechanisms of action and uses. *Hospital Practice* 1987, (Dec 15): 129–156.

Lane F (ed): Physiology of diuretic action. *Renal Physiol* 1987;10:129.

Thier Samuel O: Diuretic mechanisms as a guide to therapy. *Hospital Practice* 1987, (June 15): 81–100.

STAYING UP-TO-DATE

The most painless way for a busy clinician not specializing in nephrology to follow important developments in renal physiology is to read the excellent reviews that appear frequently in the *New England Journal of Medicine* and *Hospital Practice*. They are usually succinct and emphasize the clinical implications of new research findings. More detailed reviews are to be found in the *Annual Review of Physiology; News in Physiological Sciences (NIPS);* and the specialty journals for renal physiology, notably the *American Journal of Physiology* (renal and electrolyte section), *Kidney International, Renal Physiology,* and *Mineral and Electrolyte Metabolism.* The journals *Hypertension* and *Circulation Research* frequently have reviews on the renin-angiotensin system.

INDEX

Acetoacetate, 56
  as urinary buffer, 166
Acid, renal excretion of, 163–169
Acid-base disorders, 174–176
Acidosis, 159
  effects on potassium distribution, 141
  effects on potassium excretion, 153–154
  renal compensation for, 171
  (see also Metabolic acidosis; Respiratory acidosis)
Acids, organic (see Organic acids)
ACTH (see Adrenocorticotropic hormone)
Adenosine
  and renal hemodynamics, 82
  in tubuloglomerular feedback, 72
ADH (see Antidiuretic hormone)
Adrenal cortex, 119, 121
Adrenocorticotropic hormone, 121, 122
Afferent arterioles, 13, 14
Albumin, renal handling of, 57–58
Aldosterone, 96
  control of potassium secretion by, 145, 147–149
  control of secretion, 121–122, 123
  control of sodium reabsorption by, 119–121
  effect on tubular hydrogen-ion secretion, 173
  effects on potassium distribution, 142

Aldosterone (Cont.):
  inhibitors of, 151
  role in producing metabolic alkalosis, 178–180
  summary of controls of secretion of, 148
  summary of effects, 174
Aldosteronism (see Hyperaldosteronism)
Alkalosis, 159
  effects on potassium distribution, 141
  effects on potassium excretion, 153
  renal compensation for, 170
  tubular secretion of bicarbonate in, 163
  (see also Metabolic alkalosis; Respiratory alkalosis)
Alpha-ketoglutarate, 168
Amino acids, renal handling of, 55–57
Ammonium
  control of renal excretion of, 171–172
  synthesis and excretion of, 167–169
Angiotensin-converting enzyme, 4
Angiotensin I, 4
Angiotensin II, 4, 5
  control of ADH secretion by, 132
  control of aldosterone secretion by, 121, 122
  and control of K_f, 117–118
  direct tubular effects of, 126
  effect on renal hemodynamics, 76
  effect on renin secretion, 80

221

Angiotensin II (*Cont.*):
  effect on thirst, 137
  summary of effects, 137–138
  in tubuloglomerular feedback, 72
Angiotensin III, 5
Angiotensinogen, 4, 5
Anions, organic (*see* Organic anions)
Antidiuretic hormone
  control of renal hemodynamics by,
    81–82
  control of secretion by
    baroreceptors, 131–133
  control of secretion by
    osmoreceptors, 133–135
  effect on renin secretion, 80
  effect on urea reabsorption, 106
  effects on water reabsorpion,
    98–99, 104–105
  in secondary hyperaldosteronism,
    133
  summary of control of secretion,
    134–135
Arterial blood pressure, regulation of,
  3–5
Ascending thin limb of Henle's loop,
  11, 12
Aspirin, 64–66
ATPase, types of, 33
Atrial natriuretic factor, 127
  in congestive heart failure, 129
Atrial natriuretic peptide (*see* Atrial
  natriuretic factor)
Atriopeptin (*see* Atrial natriuretic
  factor)
Auriculin (*see* Atrial natriuretic
  factor)
Autoregulation, 69–73

Balance concept, 2
Baroreceptors
  control of ADH secretion by,
    131–133
  in control of GFR, 115–117
  in control of sodium excretion, 113,
    114
Bases, organic (*see* Organic bases)
Basolateral membrane, 35
Beta-adrenergic receptors, in control
  of renin secretion, 78–80

Beta-hydroxybutyrate, 56
  as urinary buffer, 166
Bicarbonate
  addition to plasma by kidneys,
    163–169
  addition to plasma during
    ammonium production, 168–169
  excretion of, 159–163
  filtration of, 159
  reabsorption of, 91, 161–162, 167
  renal net addition to or elimination
    from body, 169–171
  secretion of, 162–163, 210
Bidirectional transport, 42
Bilirubin, production of, 3
Blood supply, to nephron, 13–15
Bone, in calcium homeostasis,
  184–185, 186, 187, 188
Bowman's capsule, 7
  hydraulic pressure in, 30
Bowman's space, 7
Bradykinin, 17
Buffering, 158–159

Calcitonin, 188
Calcium
  concentration in plasma, 182
  effect on renin secretion, 80
  effector sites for homeostasis,
    182–185
  effects of parathyroid hormone on,
    185–187
  renal handling of, 183–184
Calyx, 6, 7
Carbonic anhydrase, 160, 161, 162
Carbonic anhydrase inhibitors, 207
Carotid sinus (*see* Baroreceptors)
Carriers, 33, 34
Cations, organic (*see* Organic cations)
Chemical messengers, intrarenal, 17
Chloride depletion, role in metabolic
  alkalosis, 177–178
Chloride reabsorption, 89–90, 92
  in collecting ducts, 96–99
  in distal convoluted tubule, 96–99
  in loop of Henle, 94–96
  in proximal tubule, 90–94
  summary of, 97
Cirrhosis, 130

Clearance, 44–54
Collecting ducts, 11, 12
  bicarbonate reabsorption in, 161,
    167
  fluid reabsorption by, 96–99
  in urine concentration, 104–105
Collecting-duct system, 11, 12–13
Colloid osmotic pressure (see Oncotic
    pressure)
Colloids, 23
Congestive heart failure, 129–130
  potassium excretion in, 150
Connecting tubule, 11, 12
Cortical collecting duct, 11, 12
  electrolyte transport by, 209
  handling of potassium by, 143,
    144–152
  potassium secretion and fluid
    delivery to, 149–151
  secretion of bicarbonate by,
    162–163
  sodium reabsorption in, 35–37
Cortisol
  effect on sodium reabsorption, 127
  effects on calcium balance, 189
Cotransport, 34
Countercurrent exchange, 106–107,
    108
Countercurrent multiplier system,
    99–108
Countertransport, 34
Creatinine
  clearance as measure of GFR, 46
  plasma concentration and GFR,
    52–54
  production of, 3
Crystalloids, 23

Descending thin limb of Henle's loop,
    11, 12
Diabetes insipidus, 135
Diabetes mellitus
  excretion of buffers in, 166
  osmotic diuresis in, 94
Diarrhea
  reflexes elicited by, 116–117
  as source of hydrogen-ion gain, 157
Diffusion, 33
1,25-Dihydroxyvitamin D_3, 5

1,25-Dihydroxyvitamin D_3 (Cont.):
  effects of, 187–188
Diluting segments, 109
Distal convoluted tubule, 11, 12
  electrolyte transport by, 209
  fluid reabsorption by, 96–99
  handling of potassium by, 143
Diuretics
  classes of, 207
  effects on potassium excretion, 151
  production of metabolic alkalosis
    by, 179–180
  and tubuloglomerular feedback, 73
Dopamine
  effect on sodium reabsorption, 127
  and renal hemodynamics, 82
Drugs, 3
  renal handling of, 67

Effective renal blood flow, 49–50
Effective renal plasma flow, 49
Efferent arterioles, 13, 14
Eicosanoids, 5, 17
  (see also Prostaglandins;
    Thromboxane)
Electrical hindrance, 24
Electrical potential difference, 89
Electrolyte transport (summary
    figures), 208–210
Endocytosis, 34
Epinephrine
  in control of GFR, 115
  control of renal hemodynamics by,
    73
  effects on potassium distribution,
    141–142
ERBF (see Effective renal blood
    flow)
ERPF (see Effective renal plasma
    flow)
Erythropoietin, 5
Estrogen, effect on sodium
    reabsorption, 127
Extracellular volume, role in
    metabolic alkalosis, 177

Facilitated diffusion, 33
Filtration coefficient, 27, 28–29
  effect of angiotensin II on, 76

Filtration coefficient (*Cont.*):
  glomerular (*see* Glomerular
    filtration coefficient)
Filtration fraction
  effect of sympathetic reflexes on,
    75
  and sodium reabsorption, 125–126
Fixed acids, 156
Food additives, 3
Foot processes, 9
Foreign chemicals, 3
Fractional excretion (FE), 51–52

Gastrointestinal tract, in calcium
    homeostasis, 183
GFR (*see* Glomerular filtration rate)
Glomerular capillary pressure, 29–30
  control of, 115–117
Glomerular filtrate, 20
  composition of, 23–24
Glomerular filtration, 20, 23–31
  barrier to macromolecules, 24
  net filtration pressure in, 24–26
Glomerular filtration coefficient,
    physiological control of, 117–118
Glomerular filtration rate, 26–31
  autoregulation of, 69–73
  control by sympathetic reflexes, 74
  control of, 115–118
  control of by ADH, 81–82
  effect of angiotensin II on, 75
  measurement of, 44–46
Glomerular membranes, 24
Glomerulotubular balance, 118–119
Glomerulus, 6
Glucagon
  effect on phosphate excretion, 189
  effect on sodium reabsorption, 127
Gluconeogenesis, 6
Glucose
  mechanism of reabsorption of,
    37–38
  quantity reabsorbed, 40
  renal handling of, 55–57
  transport maximum for, 38–40
Glutamate, 168
Glutamine
  catabolism and ammonium
    excretion, 167–169

Glutamine (*Cont.*):
  control of renal metabolism of,
    171–172
Granular cells, 16
Growth hormone
  effect on sodium reabsorption, 127
  effects on calcium balance, 189

H-ATPase, 160, 163
Hemorrhage
  oncotic pressure in, 117
  renal vasoconstriction in, 73–74
Hormones, renal handling of, 58
Hydraulic permeability, 27
Hydrogen ion
  control of tubular secretion,
    172–174
  quantitation of renal handling of,
    169–171
  renal excretion of, 163–169
  secretion and bicarbonate
    reabsorption, 160–162
  secretion by collecting duct, 167
  secretion by proximal tubule, 167
  secretion of and excretion on
    urinary buffers, 164–167
  sources of gain and loss, 156–158
Hydroxyapatite, 184
Hyperaldosteronism, 130
Hyperparathyroidism, 187
Hypocalcemic tetany, 182
Hypotension, renal vasoconstriction
    in, 74
Hypothalamus, secretion by ADH by,
    131

Inner medullary collecting duct, 11,
    12
Innervation of kidneys, 16–17
Insensible loss, 84
Insulin
  effect on phosphate excretion, 189
  effect on potassium distribution,
    142
  effect on sodium reabsorption, 127
Intercalated cells, 13
  electrolyte transport by, 209, 210
  secretion of bicarbonate by,
    162–163

Interstitial hydraulic pressure, 122–126
Intrarenal baroreceptors, 77, 78, 79
Intrarenal chemical messengers, 17
Intrarenal physical factors, 122–126
Inulin, 45–46
Isolated perfused tubule, 18

JG apparatus (see Juxtaglomerular apparatus)
Juxtaglomerular apparatus, 4, 16

Kallikrein, 17
K_f (see Filtration coefficient)
Kidneys
  functions of, 2–6
  structure of, 6–17
Kinins, 17, 18
  effect on sodium reabsorption, 127
Krebs cycle intermediates, 55

Lactate, 56
Leaky epithelia, 42–43
Lipids, vasodilators, 5
Liver, and glutamine metabolism, 169
Loop diuretics, 207
Loops of Henle, 13
  fluid reabsorption by, 100–102
  handling of potassium by, 141–142
  reabsorption of fluid by, 94–96
Luminal membrane, 35
Lysyl bradykinin, 17

Macula densa, 11, 12, 16
  in control of renin secretion, 77, 79
  in tubuloglomerular feedback, 70–73
Medullary collecting duct, 11, 12
  electrolyte transport by, 209
  handling of potassium by, 143
Mesangial cells
  effect of angiotensin II on, 118
  extraglomerular, 16
  glomerular, 10
Metabolic acidosis, 175–176
  effect on calcium excretion, 184
Metabolic alkalosis, 176
  renal generation or maintenance of, 176–180
Metabolism, by tubules, 43

Methods, in renal physiology, 17–18
Micropuncture, 17–18
Myogenic mechanism, 70

Na, H-countertransporter, 160, 163
Na, K, 2Cl cotransporter, 95
Na, K-ATPase, 36, 86
Nephron
  blood supply to, 13–15
  structure of, 6–13
Nephrons, populations of, 15
Nephrosis, 130
Net filtration pressure, in glomerular filtration, 24–26
Nonvolatile acids, 156

Obligatory water loss, 100
Oncotic pressure
  in glomerular capillaries, 30
  plasma, and GFR, 116, 117
  and sodium reabsorption, 124–125
Oral contraceptives, 5
Organic acids
  renal handling of, 64–67
  as urinary buffers, 165–167
Organic anions, renal handling of, 61–63
Organic bases, renal handling of, 64–67
Organic cations, renal handling of, 63–64
Organic substances, renal handling of, 55–67
Osmolarity, changes along proximal tubule, 91
Osmoreceptors, control of ADH secretion by, 133–135
Osmotic diuretics, 93–94
Outer medullary collecting duct, 11, 12

PAH (see Para-aminohippurate)
Papilla, 6, 7
Papillary collecting duct, 11, 12
Para-aminohippurate
  clearance as measure of ERPF, 49
  renal handling of, 61–63
Paracellular transport, 34–35
Parafollicular cells, 188

Parathyroid glands, 185
Parathyroid hormone
  control of secretion, 185–187
  effect on 1, 25-dihydroxyvitamin D_3
    production, 188
  effect on sodium reabsorption, 127
  effects, 185–187
Paraventricular nucleus, 131
P_{CO_2}, effect on tubular hydrogen
    secretion, 173
Pelvis, renal, 6, 7
Peptides, renal handling of, 58
Peritubular capillaries, 13, 14
  fluid movement into, 87–89
Peritubular capillary hydraulic
    pressure, 124–126
Pesticides, 3
pH, effect on tubular function, 66–67
Phosphate
  effects of parathyroid hormone on,
    185, 186
  reabsorption of, 166
  renal handling of, 189-190
  as urinary buffer, 164–167
Physical factors (*see* Intrarenal
    physical factors)
pK, 66–67
Podocytes, 7, 8
Potassium
  control of aldosterone secretion by,
    121, 122
  effect of diuretics on excretion, 151
  effect on renin secretion, 80
  effects of acid-base changes on
    excretion of, 153–154
  homeostatic control of excretion,
    145–149
  regulation of internal distribution,
    140–141
  renal handling of, 141–154
  tubular secretion of, 143–152
Potassium depletion, role in
    producing metabolic alkalosis,
    178–180
Potassium-sparing diuretics, 151, 207
Pregancy, and sodium reabsorption,
    127
Pressure natriuresis, 126
Primary active transport, 33

Primary hyperaldosteronism, 130,
    178–179
Principal cells, 13
  effects of aldosterone on, 120
  electrolyte transport by, 209
  secretion of potassium by, 144
Progesterone, effect on sodium
    reabsorption, 127
Prorenin, 4–5
Prostacyclin, 17
Prostaglandin E_2, 17
Prostaglandins
  and antidiuretic hormone, 98–99
  control of renal blood flow by,
    80–81
  effect on renin secretion, 80
  effect on sodium reabsorption, 128
  in tubuloglomerular feedback, 72
Protein
  filtration of, 24
  renal handling of, 57–58
Proximal tubule, 12
  bicarbonate reabsorption by,
    161–162, 167
  concentration changes along, 91
  electrolyte transport by, 208
  reabsorption of fluid by, 90–94
  reabsorption of organic anions by,
    61–63
  reabsorption of organic substances
    by, 54–56
  reabsorption of potassium by, 141
  secretion of organic cations by,
    63–64
  synthesis of ammonium by, 167–168
Pump-leak systems, 42
Pyramid, renal, 6, 7

Reabsorption (*see* Tubular
    reabsorption)
Renal blood flow
  autoregulation of, 69–73
  control by sympathetic reflexes,
    74–75
  control by ADH, 81–82
  effect of angiotensin II on, 75
  intrarenal distribution of, 82
Renal clearance (*see* Clearance)
Renal corpuscle, 6, 10

Renal cortex, 6, 7
Renal hemodynamics, control of,
    68–82
Renal medulla, 6, 7
Renal nerves (*see* Sympathetic
    nerves)
Renal pelvis, 6, 7
Renal plasma flow, effect on
    glomerular oncotic pressure, 30
Renal pyramid, 6, 7
Renin, 4–5
    control of secretion, 77–80
Renin-angiotensin system, 3–5
Reninlike proteins, 5
Respiratory acidosis, 174–175
Respiratory alkalosis, 174–175
Rickets, 188

Salt, bodily balance of, 84–85
Salt appetite, 137
Secondary active transport, 34
Secondary hyperaldosteronism,
    130–131
    and ADH, 133
Secretion (*see* Tubular secretion)
Sieving, 24
Slits, 9
Sodium
    balance and potassium secretion,
        149–151
    bodily balance of, 84–85
    control of aldosterone secretion by,
        121
    control of excretion, 113, 129
    effect on calcium excretion, 184
    quantity reabsorbed, 40
Sodium reabsorption, 85–89
    in collecting ducts, 96–99
    control of, 118–128
    in cortical collecting duct, 35–37
    in distal convoluted tubule, 96–99
    in loop of Henle, 94–96
    in proximal tubule, 90–94
    summary of, 109–110
Sodium retention, 129–131
Splay, 39
Steric hindrance, 24
Supraoptic nucleus, 131
Sweating

Sweating (*Cont.*):
    control of sodium excretion in, 136
    GFR in, 117
Sympathetic nerves
    in control of GFR, 115–117
    control of renal hemodynamics by,
        73–76
    in control of renin secretion, 78–80
    direct tubular effects of, 126
    to kidneys, 16
    renal effects of, 127
    and sodium reabsorption, 124, 125

Tetany, hypocalcemic, 182
Thiazide diuretics, 207
Thick ascending limb of Henle's loop,
    11, 12
    electrolyte transport by, 208
Thirst, 135–137
Threshold, 39
Thromboxane, 17
Tight epithelia, 42–43
Tight junctions, 34–35
Titratable acid, 170
T_m (*see* Transport maximum)
Total renal plasma flow, 49
Transcellular transport, 35
Transport maximum, 38–40, 56
Transport mechanisms, classification
    of 33–34
TRPF (*see* Total renal plasma flow)
Tubular metabolism, 43
Tubular reabsorption, 20, 31–40
    quantitation of, 50–52
    transport mechanisms in, 34–40
Tubular secretion, 20
    mechanism of, 40–42
    quantitation of, 50–52
Tubule, 6
    structure of, 10–13
Tubuloglomerular feedback, 70–73

Urate, renal handling of, 62–63
Urea
    and ammonium metabolism, 169
    clearance of, 50
    plasma concentration and GFR,
        52–54
    production of, 3

Urea (*Cont.*):
  quantity reabsorbed, 40
  renal handling of, 58–61
  role in urine concentration, 105, 106
Ureter, 7, 12
Uric acid, 3
Urinary bladder, 7, 12
Urinary space, 7
Urine concentrating mechanisms,
  99–108

Vasa recta, 14, 15
  in urine concentration, 106–107, 108
Vascular bundles, 14, 15
Vasoactive substances, 5
Vasodilator lipids, 5
Vasopressin (*see* Antidiuretic
  hormone)
Vitamin D (*see* 1,25-Dihydroxyvitamin
  D_3)

Vitamin D_3, 187
Vitamins, 56
Vomiting, as source of hydrogen-ion
  loss, 157

Waste products, renal excretion of, 3
Water
  bodily balance of, 84
  quantity reabsorbed, 40
Water reabsorption
  in collecting ducts, 96–99
  coupling to sodium reabsorption,
    87–89
  in distal convoluted tubule, 96–99
  in loop of Henle, 94–96
  in proximal tubule, 90–94
  summary of, 109–110
Weak acids and bases, 64–67

Zona glomerulosa, 120